AUTOPHAGY

How to Purify our Body, Promote Muscle Growth, Slow Aging and Prevent the Onset of Cancer through Specific and Targeted Diets!

MELANY FLORES

Copyright © 2019 by Melany Flores

All rights reserved

This book or parts thereof may not be reproduced in any form, stored in any retrieval system, or transmitted in any form by any means—electronic, mechanical, photocopy, recording, or otherwise without prior written permission of the publisher, except as provided by United States of America copyright law

CONTENTS

- INTRODUCTION 1
- THE SCIENCE BEHIND AUTOPHAGY 4
- KEY REGULATORS OF AUTOPHAGY 11
- WHAT CAN GO WRONG WITH AUTOPHAGY? 15
- ROLE OF AUTOPHAGY IN INFLAMMATION AND RELATED DISEASES 22
- THE ROLE OF AUTOPHAGY IN CANCER 29
- AUTOPHAGY AND ITS ROLE IN AGING 35
- HOW WE CAN INDUCE OR PROMOTE AUTOPHAGY 38
- ROLE OF VARIOUS DIETARY COMPONENTS IN AUTOPHAGY 51
- AUTOPHAGY AND OBESITY 81
- ROLE OF AUTOPHAGY IN INCREASING LIFESPAN 94
- ROLE OF AUTOPHAGY IN THE BODY 107
- METHODS TO MONITOR AUTOPHAGY 120
- WHEN DO THE RESULTS OF AUTOPHAGY START TO SHOW? 125
- AUTOPHAGY—THE BEST BODY DETOX REGIMEN 127
- PRECAUTIONS RELATED TO AUTOPHGY 128
- FUTURE PERSPECTIVES REGARDING AUTOPHAGY AND ITS THERAPEUTIC ROLE 130
- CONCLUSION AND FINAL THOUGHTS 133

INTRODUCTION

What is Autophagy?

The human body contains many intricate regulatory mechanisms that ensure the normal functioning of millions of cells. One such regulatory mechanism is known as autophagy. Autophagy plays a significant role in the body as it ensures the removal of old, worn-out substances, including damaged organelles, abnormal or old proteins, and cell debris. It is essentially a recycling process that occurs in all eukaryotes. It is also involved in the regulation of a variety of cellular functions, such as cell death, cell differentiation and growth, oxidative stress, the nutrient-deficiency stress response and organelle turnover.

Autophagy is a highly conserved process and is a major reliever of various stress conditions for cells. It also plays an essential role in the extension of a cell's lifespan. The term autophagy was coined by Christian de Duve about half a century ago. Since then, it has been the focus of many types of research and has helped us understand the physiological processes of cell regulation and recycling in the body.

Significance of Autophagy

Autophagy is a hallmark of energy generation processes when the cell's energy reserves are scarce and the body is in the starvation phase. The breakdown of cellular components provides energy for metabolic processes which primarily include the production of new proteins and membranes. It also provides the necessary energy for survival in stressful conditions such as starvation and nutrient deficiency. Autophagy is the main process that maintains the health of cells and organs as it replaces old and outdated components of a cell with new ones.

Autophagy affects the overall metabolic homeostasis of the body; nearly all the vital metabolic processes that occur in the body are directly or indirectly dependent on this process to function optimally. Furthermore, autophagy also plays a diverse role in the functioning of the immune system.

Types of Autophagy

There are two main types of autophagy: non-selective and selective autophagy. Selective autophagy occurs under normal conditions for the purpose of renewal and recycling of cellular components. It targets a specific substrate that needs to be removed from the cell, including damaged mitochondria, aggregates of abnormal proteins and different types of pathogens. These processes allow the removal of damaged organelles from the cell to ease the unwanted cellular burden and help to maintain the steady-state turnover of the organelles.

Selective autophagy can be further classified into different types depending on the organelle being targeted for degradation. For instance, the degradation of peroxisomes is termed pexophagy and autophagy of the mitochondria is termed mitophagy.

Non-selective autophagy occurs in cellular stress conditions, primarily when the cell faces nutrient deficiency and starvation. It does not target any specific organelle or substance and instead catabolizes random cellular components to meet the energy needs of the cell.

THE SCIENCE BEHIND AUTOPHAGY

Autophagy is a complex degradative process that involves many proteins and various pathways. Generally, this self-cannibalization mechanism is comprised of the formation of a specialized vesicle that contains abnormal and long-lived proteins and organelles in its cytoplasm. This vesicle then fuses with lysosomes that carry out the degradation process.

In this way, the cell can capture its own organelles and consume them by degrading them in the lysosome. The various benefits of autophagy have significantly increased its importance in research and studies all over the world.

Types of Autophagy According to Mechanism

Autophagy is a complex process, and it varies according to the needs of the cell and the size of the products to be degraded. Depending on the mechanism used for the transfer of organelles (cargo) to the lysosome, there are three main types of autophagy mechanisms. These include:

- Macro-autophagy
- Micro-autophagy

- Chaperone-mediated autophagy (CMA)

The mechanism of microautophagy and macroautophagy is somewhat similar as both are comprised of the dynamic rearrangement of the membrane to enclose the cytoplasm and the cargo that needs to be degraded. However, while microautophagy involves the simple engulfment of cargo at the surfaces of the lysosome by invagination and septation of the membrane of the lysosome, macroautophagy is dependent on the formation of a specialized double membraned vesicle around the cargo (the autophagosome) via *de novo* synthesis of the membrane. The autophagosome then fuses with a lysosome and empties the inner contents into the lysosome for degradation. In both cases, the membrane-bound content is degraded, and the resulting nutrients and macromolecules are transported back into the cytosol to be utilized for various metabolic processes.

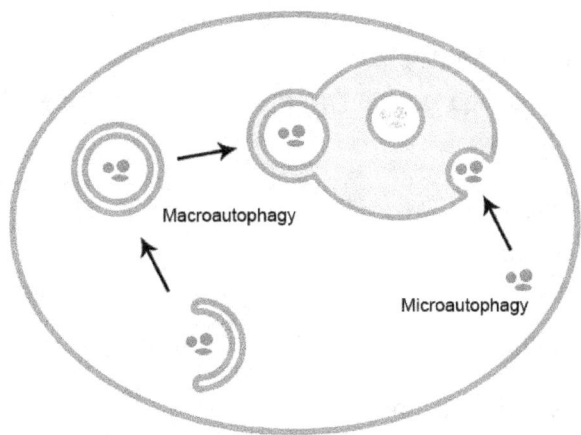

Figure 1. Types of autophagy.

The third type of autophagy does not involve any special membrane arrangements or the formation of a vesicle. Instead, it uses specific chaperones that directly transfer abnormally formed proteins and other cargo across the membrane of lysosome for degradation.

The most common and most widely understood autophagy is macroautophagy. Most published studies have focused on macroautophagy; this book will also be focusing on macroautophagy to avoid confusion and help us better understand the process and its effects on our body.

Mechanism of Macroautophagy

Autophagy involves the formation of a specific cavity or vesicle that engulfs or surround the substances that need to be degraded. This membrane-bound structure then fuses with the lysosome and transfer its contents, termed as cargo, into it for degradation. This process involves the role of around 16 different proteins that ensure the proper execution of autophagy. The complete process of autophagy can be divided into seven distinct steps. These are given below:

- Induction
- Nucleation
- Expansion and recognition of cargo
- Recycling of proteins
- Fusion of vesicle with the lysosome

- Digestion
- Recycling of cargo

Formation of Autophagosome

The primary step in the process of autophagy is the production of autophagosome or the vesicle. Around sixteen different Atg proteins control the formation of the autophagosome. The average diameter of the autophagosome is approximately 0.9 μm in yeast and about 1.5 μm in mammals. Various environmental cues, such as nutrient deficiency, are picked up by cell receptors such as mTORC1 that become inactive and cause the activation of the ULK1 complex that then affects the activity of P13K complex. This complex plays a central role in the early stages of the formation of the autophagosome by mediating the production of the phagophore from which the isolation membrane of autophagosome originates. Various Atg proteins including Atg-12, Atg-9, Atg-5 and Atg16L1 play a critical role in the elongation of isolation membrane.

In the next step, the autophagosome fuses with the cell vesicles (derived from the endosome) and forms a structure known as amphisome. This structure combines with the lysosome to form the autolysosome. When the components of the autophagosome are transferred to the lysosome, they are attacked by hydrolases and degraded into smaller molecules. These molecules help to replenish the energy and metabolic needs of the body, and the signal of the presence of a high level of nutrients reactivate the mTORC1 that leads to the suppression of autophagy.

Stepwise Process of Autophagy

The primary step in the process of autophagy, where the production of autophagosome occurs, is termed as induction or initiation. In this step, the membrane of the cell begins to expand and forms the phagophore, which is a double membrane sequestering compartment. This membrane expands to form the spherical autophagosome and wraps itself around the cargo. At this stage, the LC3-II is cleaved from the outer part of this double-membraned structure. The autophagosome then finds the lysosome, and its outer membrane fuses with the lysosomal membrane to form a structure known as the autolysosome.

However, in some cases, the autophagosome fuses with an endosome and forms a specialized structure known as the amphisome before it reaches and fuses with a lysosome.

The cargo is delivered from the autophagosome to the lysosome and is degraded and exported back into the cytoplasm through lysosomal channels known as permeases. The products of autophagy are reused for various processes in the cell.

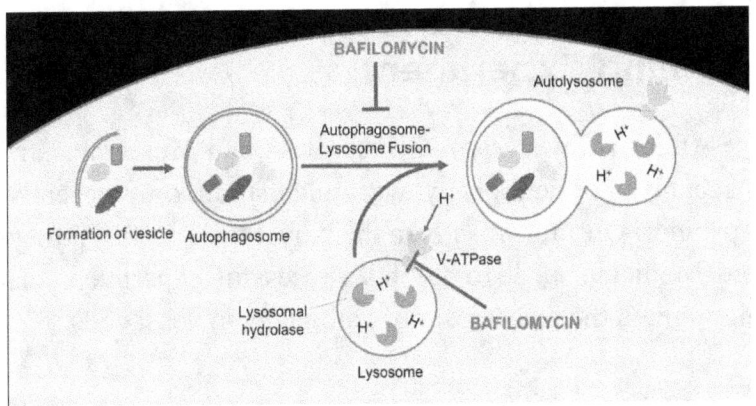

Figure 2. Formation of autophagosome.

Genetics of Autophagy

Several genome-wide studies have highlighted the role of various genes in the process of autophagy. These autophagy-related genes are marked as ATG genes and are involved in multiple cellular processes of autophagy. These genes were initially identified in yeast, and various studies suggest that there is conservation of autophagy machinery among all eukaryotes. Various orthologs of ATG genes of yeast have also been found to be present in various higher organisms.

In yeast, the induction of the autophagosome is regulated by the Atg1-Atg13-Atg17-Atg31-Atg29 kinase complex. In mammals, the autophagosome is formed by a homolog of Atg1 ULK1 or ULK2, Atg13, RB1-inducible coiled-coil 1 (RB1CC1/FIP200) and C12orf44/ATG101. This complex (ULK1/2-ATG13-RB1CC1) will carry out autophagy regardless of the nutrient status of the cells.

Melany Flores

Autophagy and the Nobel Prize-Winning Experiment

After many years of studies and research, the mechanism of autophagy was understood only recently. Yoshinori Ohsumi was given the Nobel Prize in Physiology and Medicine in 2016 for his successful experiment that highlighted the mechanism of autophagy in yeast cells.

KEY REGULATORS OF AUTOPHAGY

Autophagy is a naturally occurring process in the body that is primarily induced in response to various environmental and physiological stress factors. Some environmental factors are deprivation of food, deprivation of oxygen and exposure to high temperatures. The most significant physiological factor of induction of autophagy is aging. Moreover, the relationship between autophagy and aging also shares a remarkable interaction at the molecular level.

Nutrient homeostasis maintains the physiological functions of the cells. Autophagy is a highly efficient process that carries out the recycling of the nutrients in the body and thus maintains the nutrient homeostasis. The process of autophagy is activated when cells undergo nutritional stress, which include nutrient deficiency (starvation) or nutrient excess. Two protein kinases, AMP-activated protein kinase and the mammalian target of rapamycin (mTOR), regulate the process of autophagy. These enzymes monitor the energy and amino acids levels in the cell. When autophagy is activated in starvation conditions, the damaged organelles and proteins are degraded and the nutrient status of the cell is replenished. However, uncontrolled or unnecessary induction of autophagy can lead to cell death. Thus, the equilibrium between the induction and suppression of autophagy is crucial for determining the fate of the cell. Nutrient excess can also lead to autophagy.

There are three main kinases that carry out the regulation of macroautophagy at the cellular level. These kinases act as sensors and read the environmental and physiological signals that lead to the induction of autophagy. They include AMP-activated protein kinases (AMPK), mechanistic target of rapamycin complex1 (MTORC1) and cAMP- activated protein kinase (PKA).

Relationship Between Autophagy, Cellular Energy Levels, and Starvation

In the 1970s, various researchers established a definite relationship between the nutritional status of a cell and autophagy. Starvation was identified as the first stimulus that led to the activation of autophagy. The benefits of the process of autophagy in starved cells were quite clear as it played a central role in the energy homeostasis of the cell by recycling cellular components and amino acids through catabolic action of lysosomes.

Autophagy carries out catabolism of different essential nutrients of the diet. When there is a depletion of nutrients, autophagy ensures the survival of the cell by carrying out the degradation of intracellular proteins to provide essential amino acids. These amino acids can be used in the synthesis of proteins or can directly enter the Krebs's cycle for the generation of energy currency, i.e., ATP. The presence of nutrients and the replenishing of cellular energy levels lead to the suppression of autophagy. In this way, autophagy is a self-regulated process which is highly sensitive to the energy markers of the cells.

Another role of autophagy in the maintenance of energy levels and nutrient pools of the cell is that it functions to mobilize the intracellular lipid stores and glycogen reserves to generate energy during the period of starvation. The breakdown of intracellular stores of nutrients by macroautophagy can also occur when there are high levels of glucose and fats in the cells. This mechanism helps the cell to manage the size of intracellular stores and avoids nutrient burdening of the cell.

There are special nutrient sensors that help medicate the process of autophagy in the cell. These sensors provide the required communication between the nutritional status of the cell and autophagy. The essential mammalian sensor of nutritional status that also regulates the process of macroautophagy is the mammalian target of rapamycin (mTOR). These enzymes read nutritional cues such as the presence of amino acids, ATP levels, and insulin in the body and upregulate or downregulate the process of autophagy accordingly.

Starvation that is primarily marked by reduced levels of nutrients and insulin in the body that leads to the inactivation of mTOR through the influence of AMP-activated protein kinase (AMPK) is another cellular nutrient sensor. Inactivation of mTOR leads to the production of the autophagy initiation complex and the formation of autophagosomes.

WHAT CAN GO WRONG WITH AUTOPHAGY?

Autophagy is the double-edged sword in the human body.

Autophagy is a highly regulated process, and its degradative abilities make its regulation an essential entity. Any kind of errors and mutations in the genes or proteins involved in this pathway can have deleterious effects on the cells. Defects in autophagy have been found to be linked with various diseases and disorders, and this indicates the physiological significance of this process in the body. These processes include cellular differentiation, homeostasis, growth and development, and starvation.

Various studies have identified mutations in the ATG genes to be the underlying cause of multiple diseases in human, which include infectious diseases, neurodegenerative diseases and different types of cancers.

A list of diseases and their associated mutation in ATG and other genes related to autophagy are given in Table 1.

Table 1. The link between various autophagy-related genetic disorders and diseases

Sr #	Stage in Autophagy process	Gene Involved	Disease in Humans
1	Formation of autophagosome	ATG16L1	Crohn's disease
2	Formation of autophagosome	ATG5	Asthma and Lupus
3	Formation of autophagosome	EI24/PIG8	Breast Cancer
4	Formation of autophagosome	BECN1	Prostate, ovarian and colorectal cancer
5	Maturation of autophagosome	SPG15	Hereditary spastic paraparesis type 15
6	Induction of mitophagy (autophagy of mitochondria)	PARK6/PINK1	Parkinson's disease

Apart from genetic defects, malfunctioning of autophagy can have deleterious effects on the body. These include various kinds of cancer, muscular disorders, liver disease, neurodegeneration and recurrent pathogenic infections. Therefore, autophagy is a double-edged sword that can benefit or harm the cell in different conditions. The beneficial and harmful role of autophagy in the human body and how it can act in both ways is summarized in **Table 2**.

Table 2. The positive and negative effects of autophagy in the body

Disease	Positive effects of autophagy	Negative effects of autophagy
Cancer	Functions as a tumor suppressor and removes damaged organelles that could generate free radicals and increase chances of	Promotes the survival of cancer cells inside a tumor where there is deficiency of nutrients. It can protect the cancer cells from cell death, and hinders chemotherapeutic methods

	mutations	
Liver disease	Removes damaged endoplasmic reticulum	Excessive mitochondrial autophagy can lead to tissue damage
Muscular disorder	Decreases the effects of lysosomal disease	Increased autophagy and accumulation of autophagosomes leads to defects in cell function
Neurodegeneration	Removes toxic aggregates of protein	May trigger death of neurons that carry aggregated proteins
Pathogen infection	Provides protection against viruses and bacteria	Can allow pathogens to survive and grow, and provides nutrients for their growth

Role of Autophagy in Various Diseases

Autophagy and Cancer

Abnormal growth and death of cells are the hallmarks of cancer. This feature suggests a specific role of autophagy-related proteins in the triggering and progression of cancer. Autophagy keeps a check in the abnormality of components of the cell and can be considered to be a quality control center. The failure of the process of autophagy can lead to the unsuccessful degradation and removal of abnormal cells that can lead to carcinogenesis.

Various ATG genes, including the ATG5, ATG2, ATG12 ABD and UVRAG genes, have been found to be linked with several types of cancers and have been affected with microsatellite instability and point mutations. The relationship between autophagy and cancer has been an area of interest and many oncology-related studies are now focusing on the therapeutic role of the autophagy-related gene in cancer.

The autophagy gene Beclin-1 that is involved in the early stages of autophagosome formation is a tumor suppressor gene. Autophagy can kill tumor cells by removing damaged mitochondria and other abnormal organelles. Similarly, PTEN and p53 are bona fide tumor suppressor genes that can also induce autophagy in the cells. Thus, autophagy has a protective effect against cancer progression as it promotes the growth of healthy cells and destroys the abnormal cancerous cells.

Autophagy and Neurodegenerative Diseases

Various single-gene mutations linked with many multisystem disorders in children have been found to be reported in autophagy genes. These inborn errors in the autophagy system predominantly affect the health and development of the central nervous system. They have been associated with causing epilepsy, malformation of the brain, intellectual disability delay in development, neurodegeneration, and disorder of movement.

These mutations affect the various stages of autophagy and lead to a wide class of disorders termed as congenital disorders of autophagy that are part of another diverse group of disorders known as inborn errors of metabolism.

Autophagy and Inflammatory disease

There is emerging evidence that defects in autophagy play an essential role in the triggering and progression of various acute and chronic inflammatory diseases. These include Crohn's disease, pulmonary hypertension, infectious diseases, inflammatory bowel disease, cystic fibrosis, lupus, and diabetes. Autophagy impacts the regulation of various inflammatory diseases by several mechanisms. These include:

- A xenophagic response initiated by autophagy where it directly participates in the clearance of bacteria by capturing and delivering the bacteria to the lysosome for degradation.

- Autophagic assists in antigen presentation by digesting the invading pathogens.

- Various proteins involved in autophagy play an essential role in controlling many proinflammatory responses, such as the production of proinflammatory cytokines and the maintenance of the quality of mitochondrial function.

- Autophagic degradation of toxic aggregates of proteins plays a protective role in tissues. Otherwise, serious diseases such as cystic fibrosis can occur.

Role of Autophagy in Inflammation and Related Diseases

Autophagy is a multidimensional process and the association between autophagy and the inflammatory response of the body is rather complex. There are various studies that suggest that autophagy controls the development and survival of the inflammatory machinery and thus orchestrates the inflammatory response. The cells of the inflammatory machinery that are directly regulated by the process of autophagy include lymphocytes, neutrophils, and macrophages. These cells are involved in the development as well as pathogenesis of inflammation in tissues and organs. Recent evidence indicates that autophagy plays a critical role in acute and chronic inflammatory processes. This role potentially impacts the pathogenesis and progression of various inflammatory diseases.

Macrophages

Macrophages are a significant part of our defense system and can destroy pathogens by producing inflammatory cytokines, or by uptake and intracellular destruction. There is growing evidence that suggests that upregulation of autophagy leads to increased killing of ingested pathogens in macrophages. Mice with defective autophagy systems in neutrophils and macrophages tend to be more prone to infections from intracellular pathogens such as *L. monocytogenes* and *T. gondii*.

Autophagy also acts as a regulator of inflammatory process by keeping the population of macrophages in the body in check. It has been reported that autophagy is induced in several activated macrophages when exposed to oxidative stress in the form of reactive oxygen species (ROS) causing an increase in autophagosomes that lead to the death and removal of these macrophages. This can be helpful in controlling the level of inflammation in the tissues.

Neutrophils

Neutrophils are multifunctional cells of the immune system. They play a central role in the innate immune system. The presence of inflammation in tissues recruits neutrophils to the site of infection. Neutrophils then engulf the microorganism and render it inactive by fusing it with phagosomes, resulting in the formation of phagolysosomes. Inside the phagolysosomes, the action of ROS and antimicrobial peptides lead to the destruction and clearance of pathogens. The apoptosis of neutrophils leads to a decrease in inflammation. Autophagy occurs in neutrophils in both phagocytosis-dependent and independent manners. The most widely studied function of autophagy involves its role in neutrophil death, which governs the level of inflammation in the body.

Lymphocytes

Autophagy plays an important role in both innate and adaptive immune responses. These immune responses include the homeostasis of the immune system and presentation of antigens. There exists a complex and crucial relationship between T lymphocytes and autophagy. The activation of the T cell receptor (TCR) is a strong trigger for autophagy in T lymphocytes. Several autophagy-related genes are involved in the proliferation of T cells. It has been found that T lymphocytes with defective Atg3, Atg5 and Atg7 genes have decreased proliferation rates and increased rates of cell death. Autophagy plays an important role in the homeostasis of T cells; it mediates the selection of thymocytes (lymphocytes that are present in the thymus gland) and regulates their functions. Autophagic defects in thymocytes have been linked with various autoimmune diseases. Moreover, absence of autophagy leads to the accumulation of toxic reactive oxygen species in the lymphocytes which can lead to various physiological complications. The Beclin-1 gene has been found to be involved in the development of lymphocytes and proves that a critical relationship exists between autophagy and apoptosis.

Autophagy has a direct role in mediating antigen presentation to antigen-specific T cells. This process is crucial for the induction of the acquired immune response in the body. The molecules of MHC class II have been found to localize on autophagosomes. The presentation of antigens, both viral and self, by MHC class II molecules to antigen-specific CD4+ T cells is regulated by autophagic machinery. When the body is infected with a certain virus, for instance, the human simplex virus 1, the autophagic machinery regulates the MHC class I-dependent presentation of viral antigens to CD8+ T cells.

Apart from T lymphocytes, the Atg5 gene has been found to be crucial for the growth and development of B lymphocytes. Various studies suggest that Atg5 genes play an important role in the certain differentiation stages of B cells.

Crohn's Disease

Crohn's disease (CD) is a chronic disease that affects the bowel. It is characterized by inflammation, ulceration, and neutrophil influx in the upper layer of the intestine. Various environmental and genetic factors have been linked with CD. Recent studies have also found links between CD and genes that are associated with autophagy. These genes include ATG16L, and NOD2. The NOD2 protein functions as an intracellular sensor or detector of bacteria. It has the ability to induce autophagy in the intestinal cells when detecting peptidoglycan present in bacterial cell walls. Various studies in humans suggest that three NOD2 variants are associated with CD. These variants lead to loss of function of NOD2 and may contribute to the pathogenesis of CD. Moreover, a variant of the ATG16lL gene, which is involved in the synthesis of autophagosome formation, has been found to be a major risk factor for CD.

Infectious Disease

Autophagy plays a crucial role in the immune system as it can exert various anti-pathogen and anti-bacterial functions. These features tend to impart beneficial features to the autophagic process in various infectious diseases.

For instance, in the case of a *Mycobacterium tuberculosis* infection, the autophagy pathway plays a crucial role in rendering resistance against various bacterial, viral and protozoan infections. Mycobacterium tuberculosis is an intracellular parasite and dwells within cells. It can survive within phagosomes by interfering with the synthesis of phagolysosome. By promoting autophagy, the cell can get rid of the pathogen and can provide protection for the body from various infections. The role of autophagy in providing defense against other microbial pathogens including *Legionella pneumophila* and *Shigella* has also been reported.

Pulmonary Hypertension

Pulmonary arterial hypertension (PAH) is a complex disease. It is characterized by vasoconstriction, the thickening of the artery, and increase in pulmonary artery pressure. The decrease in oxygen levels in the lungs lead to the induction of autophagy which lead to damage and fibrosis of the artery.

Cystic Fibrosis

Cystic fibrosis (CF) is a disease of lungs and airways and is characterized by an inflammation of airways, accumulation of mucous in the airways, and absence of mucociliary clearance, primarily due to the mutation of a certain protein termed as cystic fibrosis transmembrane conductance regulator (CFTR).

It has been recently found that the mutation in the CFTR gene is linked with an abnormal autophagic response. The CFTR defect and autophagy deficiency together lead to the accumulation of aggregates of protein in the pulmonary tissues and inflammation of the lung.

Chronic Obstructive Pulmonary Disease

Chronic obstructive pulmonary disease (COPD) is a lung disease characterized by chronic airway inflammation and lung damage. Macroautophagy plays a complex role in the pathogenesis of COPD. Elevated levels of the LC3b-II protein have been found in blood samples of COPD patients when compared with non-COPD controls. The level of LC3b-II correlates to the over function of autophagy in the lung cells.

Genetic mutations in two macroautophagy pathway members, Beclin-1 and LC3b, have been found to be associated with a reduction in the rate of cell death in lung cells which are exposed to cigarette smoke. Furthermore, there was an inhibition of macroautophagic flux in macrophages from COPD tissues, which may contribute to inflammation in lungs and air passages.

Other systemic inflammatory diseases

There are other systemic inflammatory diseases that have been found to be associated with autophagic defects. For instance, studies show that polymorphisms in the autophagy gene Atg5can lead to increased susceptibility of systemic lupus erythematosus (SLE). SLE is a heterogenous disease caused by an autoimmune response that targets the self-antigens of the dying cells. This anomaly results in the destruction of tissues and organs by our own immune system and the driving force behind it is the defective autophagy process. Other defects in autophagy have been linked to several inflammation-associated metabolic disorders including obesity and diabetes.

The Role of Autophagy in Cancer

Autophagy playsa dual role in cancer biology as it can regulate cancer promotion and suppression. This dual role highlights the importance of autophagy in the body and categorizes it as a double-edged sword of human physiology. Under certain physiological conditions, autophagy acts as a tumor suppressor and protects the cell from the progression and survival of cancerous cells. Under different physiological conditions, autophagy helps to promote the progression and growth of cancer cells and protects them from apoptosis. Due to this, some anticancer drugs that directly regulate autophagy have been developed. Such autophagy-based chemotherapy can be used in cancer-cell destruction or survival.

It is known that autophagy regulation in the body influences the expression of tumor promotor genes (oncogenes) or tumor suppressor proteins. The factors that are involved in the suppression of tumors are negatively regulated by mTOR and AMPK. This leads to the induction of autophagy and suppresses the initiation of cancer. On the other hand, oncogenes are activated by mTOR and AKT, which is associated with the suppression of autophagy and promotes the progression of cancer. In this way, the underlying pathways that regulate autophagy indirectly decide the fate of cancerous cells in the body.

Autophagy also plays a direct role in the promotion of cancer. Abnormal autophagy processes lead to a decrease in the degradation of old and damaged organelles and proteins in cells with increased oxidative stress. This leads to the development of cancer.

Primarily, the basal process of autophagy suppresses cancer. The mutation of autophagic proteins lead to an increased risk of various types of cancers. For instance, BIF-1 proteins that are associated with BECN1 have been found to be anomalous in colorectal and stomach cancer. Similarly, the UVRAG proteins that are associated with BECN1 function as a major regulator of autophagy, and the presence of mutated UVRAG leads to a reduction in the process of autophagy, resulting inan increased proliferation rate of colorectal cancer cells.

Conversely, the tumor promoter rule of autophagy highlights the fact that high cellular levels of autophagy are linked with different types of RAS-activated cancers including pancreatic cancers. This implies that methods to suppress autophagy lead to a decrease in the proliferation of cancerous cells which improves tumor suppression.

Hence, autophagy regulates tumor initiation and suppression. The diverse roles of autophagy as an inducer of cancer and as a tumor suppressor are discussed in the sections below and summarized in Table 3.

Autophagy as a Regulator of Tumor Suppression

The intrinsic ability of autophagy to remove abnormal proteins and to degrade dysfunctional organelles and maintain the cellular homeostasis makes it a diehard tumor suppressor. The presence of any kind of mutation in autophagic genes or any metabolic error related to the physiological function of autophagy results in deleterious effects on the cell. These effects may manifest themselves in form of various metabolic disorders and cancers of various parts including the ovaries, breasts and prostate.

Various studies suggest that the autophagy mutation of the BECN gene that encodes Beclin-1, which is an important part of autophagic machinery, can appear clinically in various forms of cancer. Beclin-1 is a tumor suppressor gene as it promotes the autophagy process by the synthesis of autophagosomes. Mutations in this gene lead to increased proliferation of cancer cells as the process of autophagy that keeps a check on the cellular quality has become compromised. A decrease in cellular Beclin-1 level has also been observed in cases of other cancers, including cervical squamous-cell carcinomas and hepatocellular cancers.

There is experimental evidence that suggests that the mutation of certain other autophagic genes can also lead to tumor suppression. Certain proteins, such as UV radiation resistance-associated gene (UVRAG) function as tumor suppressor genes. Under normal conditions, it acts as a positive regulator of autophagy. The decrease in UVRAG causes an impaired autophagosome development and a decreased level of cellular autophagy. This results in an increase in cancer cell proliferation of different types of cancers, including colon, stomach, breast, and prostate cancers.

Knockout studies involving core autophagic proteins have been carried out to study the cancer-suppression role of autophagy in mice. It was found that the knockout of ATG5 and ATG7 genes from hepatocytes resulted in liver cancers. The reason behind the appearance of this major pathology was that the liver cells were unable to clear themselves from damaged mitochondria and protect themselves from oxidative stress. Autophagy prevents the cell from tumor generation by regulating the levels of reactive oxygen species (ROS). Mitochondrial damage produces excessive ROS, which is one of the major triggers of carcinogenesis. Autophagy functions to protect the cell from various stresses, and impaired autophagy has catastrophic effects on cell function and quality, and they then progress as defective cancerous cells. Similar results have been obtained by studying cell lines that are deficient of autophagic regulators, such as ATG3, ATG5 and ATG9. These findings highlight the critical role of autophagy in tumor suppression; impaired autophagy can therefore lead to oncogenesis.

Autophagy as a Regulators of Tumor Promotion

The other role of autophagy in cancer is of tumor promotion. Various studies indicate that the process of autophagy promotes the survival of cancer cells and aids in the progression of tumors in later or advanced stages of cancer. So, autophagy acts as a tumor suppressor and tries to stop the progression of cancer in early stages, but if it fails due to any reason and the cancer spreads and reaches the metastasis stage, autophagy aids the tumor cells in surviving and developing.

The cells inside tumors suffer from various stresses, including low oxygen levels and poor availability of nutrients. Autophagy plays an intrinsic role in aiding the tumor cells in surviving these stresses. It also leads to the activation of autophagy in the central part of tumors where cells are exposed to extreme hypoxic conditions. The decrease in cellular autophagy due to the deletion of Beclin-1 increases cell death in tumors as the hypoxic and nutrient deficient cells are no longer protected by autophagy.

In addition to providing protection against the oxidative stresses of tumor cells, autophagy provides energy to proliferating tumors. It carries out the recycling of intracellular organelles and components and fulfills the metabolic needs of the growing tumor cells.

In animal models with impaired autophagy processes, tumor cells have been observed to undergo metabolic stress which leads to the decreased survival of cancer cells. In this way, autophagy plays a central role in the survival of tumor cells by improving their stress tolerance and by supplying the cells with necessary nutrients to meet their metabolic demands. Without these tumor-protective effects of autophagy as observed in knockout or knockdown animal models of autophagy, there is an increased rate of tumor cell death.

Table 3. Dual role of autophagy in cancer

Sr #	Autophagy induction under stress conditions in cancer cells	
	Tumor Suppressor Effects	*Tumor Promotor Effects*
1	Inhibits the growth of the tumor	Aids tumor cells to overcome various stresses
2	Maintains the homeostasis of the cell	Provides tumor cells with the required metabolic energy
3	Provides protection against cellular stresses	Degrades damaged organelles
4	Decreases the formation of tumor	Favors the formation of tumor by not removing oxidative stress

Autophagy and its Role In Aging

Autophagy is the renewal system of the cell. The more efficient the system is, the more replenished and rejuvenated the cells and organs become. This effect of autophagy on the revitalization of the human system suggests its direct role in human aging. Various studies have found that there is a definite genetic link between the genes of autophagy and the aging process.

There is a decrease in the efficiency of autophagy with age, and these findings have been extensively investigated in the yeast system. Mutants that carry defects in macroautophagy related genes have a shorter lifespan as compared to control organisms. Similarly, in nematodes, for example *Caenorhabditis elegans*, the mutants carrying a loss of function mutation in Atg1, Atg7 and Beclin-1 showed a significant decrease in their lifespan as compared to normal samples. The knockout studies of autophagy-related genes in other organisms, including fruit fly and murine models highlight the importance of the autophagy process in aging and allowing for longer lifespans.

As mentioned before, autophagy is the quality control center of the body. As we age, autophagy loses its efficiency, and there is a progressive loss in the quality of organs function – this is also the primary indication of aging. As the function of autophagy wanes off, various age-associated pathologies start to manifest themselves. The accumulation of different toxic and abnormal organelles and proteins in the cell further aid the triggering of age-related problems, such as a reduction in muscle mass, cardiac malfunction, accumulation of lipids and cholesterol, memory loss and neurodegeneration and insulin insensitivity.

Certain other factors related to autophagy also play a vital role in the process of aging. For instance, there is a loss of genomic maintenance by autophagy due to the aging process. Oxidative stress that can harm the DNA structure and its integrity is significantly reduced by autophagic actions, and various studies also suggest that there is a definitive role of autophagy in cell cycle progression and in DNA repair systems. All these processes ensure the genomic maintenance that is equivalent to an error-free, high-functioning genome as present in a young individual. This genomic maintenance is gradually lost with aging.

Autophagy Immunosenescence and Aging

As we age, there is a gradual decrease in the activity of autophagic processes, it even becomes defective in elder humans. For instance, in old livers, the efficiency of glucagon metabolism is affected by the reduction in the process of autophagy. Autophagy and aging are interrelated, and it can be said that increasing age leads to a decrease in autophagy; this decrease can lead to early signs of aging and a short lifespan.

Genetic evidence to highlight the role of autophagy in longevity is present as the loss of macroautophagy reduces the lifespan in worms that carry defective autophagy genes. Moreover, the upregulation of macroautophagy was found in the period of life extension in almost all the experimental models. Similar findings have been reported in flies where there is an increase in age-related diseases with the suppression of autophagy genes.

The defects in the energetic balance of the body as we age are related to a decrease in efficiency of autophagy. Lack of induction of macroautophagy in response to nutritional fluctuations, such as starvation, reduce mobilization of intracellular energy stores and cause loss of protein synthesis through the recycling of amino acids.

Further, a decrease in the autophagy function makes the cells more susceptible to the toxicity of lipid accumulation. The lipid content of cells and tissues is increased with increasing age, and this has a negative effect on the functioning of autophagy. The primary reason behind this is that the lipid content of the cell is crucial for the lipid composition of autophagosomes and related organelles that play a role in the normal function of autophagy. A high level of lipids disrupts the integrity and function of vesicles and lysosomes, thus leading to loss of autophagy in older cells.

HOW WE CAN INDUCE OR PROMOTE AUTOPHAGY

Autophagy is a natural process, but there are specific ways through which it can be induced in the body and one can benefit from the positive effects of autophagy. Some of the most researched and beneficial ways to induce autophagy are given below:

1. Calorie restriction
   - Keto diet
   - Fasting
   - Protein restriction
2. Exercise and high-intensity training
3. Consumption of autophagy-promoting food and supplements
   - Coffee
   - Extra virgin olive oil
   - Turmeric
   - Supplements
4. Quality Sleep

Calorie Restriction and Autophagy

We are what we eat

Diet has been considered as the most vital factor in governing the health and longevity of humans. Adopting a healthy lifestyle that is comprised of a well-balanced diet and exercise are regarded as the key to good living. In 1935, the concept of calorie restriction (CR) gained remarkable popularity in the field of healthy eating. It was proposed that CR is the most useful dietary intervention that can positively affect longevity and increase lifespan. CR involves a considerable restriction in the intake of calories and lies between the two extremes of food consumption: extremely low food consumption that can lead to starvation and death and extremely high food consumption that can lead to obesity.

There are two main practices of calorie restriction: the keto diet and intermittent fasting. Both these approaches are becoming very popular in health-conscious and/or obese individuals who want to lose weight and become fit. Obesity has become one of the leading causes of a poor lifestyle and a decreased lifespan. The keto diet and intermittent fasting can both play important roles in fighting obesity, and both share a common mechanism of action to improve quality of life, i.e., autophagy.

Mechanism of Anti-Aging Effects of Calorie Restriction

The primary anti-aging effects that result from a controlled diet are due to the role of nutrition in controlling oxidative stress as well as maintaining the genomic and mitochondrial DNA repair mechanism, the concentration of peroxide lipids and protein carbonyls in the tissues and membrane fluidity and functionality. As we age, the oxidative stress in the body is increased while the DNA repair mechanism becomes less efficient and the membrane of the cell loses its fluidity and functionality. However, autophagy is the process that can significantly reduce and reverse these effects of aging as it can influence all these processes.

Selecting the right diet and keeping a check on what we eat is a very critical factor in achieving a long and healthy life. Interestingly, all the signs of aging described above can be regulated by autophagy and related pathways. For instance, calorie restriction has a direct role in suppressing the target of rapamycin (mTOR) which leads to the promotion of autophagy and provides protection against bone disease, motor dysfunction, immune disorders, and insulin sensitivity. CR also decreases the production of IGF-1, which is the primary metabolic intervention that provides protection against age-related diseases and extends one's lifespan. When AMPK is activated, it leads to the downregulation of mTOR and subsequent activation of autophagy. The FOXO gene is also activated by the upregulation of genes related to autophagy and DNA repair, and downregulated by genes that control proliferation and growth of the cell.

Moreover, a nutrient-rich and calorie-restricted diet directly mediates anti-aging effects through upregulation of autophagy. Autophagy functions to provide protection against oxidative stress and eliminates damaged cells and aged organelles from the cell. This allows the cell to become free from unnecessary burdens, dysfunctions, and premature cell death. Autophagy removes the signs of aging from the cell and provides structural and metabolic integrity to it. Various studies suggest that calorie restriction is the most potent inducer of autophagy and has a crucial role in the prevention of age-related diseases.

Keto diet and Autophagia

The trick that makes your body eat your own fat and help you age backwards

What is the keto diet?

The intake of a high-fat diet that is comprised of polyunsaturated fatty acids is termed as the keto diet. The keto diet has a very low intake of carbohydrates, with a fat to carbohydrate ratio of around 5:1.

How does it work?

The keto diet mimics the natural effect of starvation in the body. Ketosis is a natural process that occurs in the human body during lactation and fasting. During ketosis, the body utilizes fats as the primary source of energy instead of carbohydrates through incomplete oxidation of fatty acids. This process occurs in the liver and leads to an increase in the level of acetoacetate and hydroxybutyrate in the body - these are the end products of ketosis.

<u>How ketosis and autophagy are linked?</u>

As the keto diet induces the effects of starvation in the body, it also leads to the induction of autophagy.

Benefits of the Keto Diet

The keto diet has been linked to various health benefits other than the combating of obesity. It has significant neuroprotective effects as this diet leads to an increase in the activity of hypoxia-inducible factor-1α (HIF-1α) and decreased activity of mTORC1 in the hippocampus that leads to the induction of macroautophagy in neurons. Neuronal autophagy has preventive effects on the nervous system against neurodegenerative disorders. Autophagy also leads to the removal of damaged mitochondria that may cause oxidative stress by producing superoxides. It can also remove other protein aggregates that can deteriorate the health of the brain and nervous system. Therefore, through the process of autophagy, the keto diet helps to protect the body against serious conditions like Parkinson's disease, Alzheimer's disease and epilepsy .

Other benefits of a keto diet on the body include:

- Protection against various metabolic syndromes, prediabetes and type 2 diabetes through the loss of fat. It also helps in improving insulin sensitivity.

- Provides protective effects against various heart diseases and ensures the vascular health of an individual.

- Provides protection against cancer, which is attributed to the anti-cancer effects of autophagy.

- Induces autophagy that greatly improves the immune system and helps the body to cope with injuries and diseases in a much better way.

- Improve conditions like polycystic ovary syndrome and acne as both are related to high insulin levels and intake of sugar.

However, for most people it might not be easy to stick to a ketogenic diet for long periods of time, which is why it is essential to find alternative strategies to gain the neuroprotective and other beneficial effects of the keto diet.

Such strategies may include ingestion of coconut oil or other medium-chain triglycerides, intermittent fasting, and the use of supplements that promote ketogenesis, such as carnitine, along with dietary routines that include fasting and cutting down on the intake of carbohydrates. These alternative approaches to promote autophagy in the body are discussed in the next section.

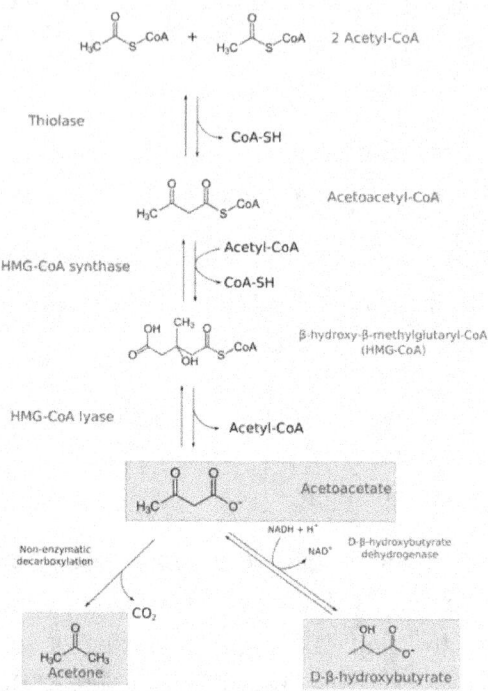

Figure 3. Ketogenesis

Fasting

Fasting is characterized by complete or partial restriction of solid food or water or both for a definite time period. Based on the duration, fasting can be of two types:

- Intermittent fasting (IF) that is characterized by alternate-day fasting of around ≥16 hours or 48 hours of fasting per week.

- Periodic fasting (PF) that is characterized by a minimum of 3 days of fasting in a bi-monthly pattern.

Role of Fasting in Promoting the Anti-Cancer Effects of Autophagy

Fasting has an extraordinary healing effect on the body and has been recognized as one of the most beneficial lifestyle choices that can detox the body and help the rejuvenation of cells and organs. The role of fasting in the induction of autophagy can be considered as a critical feature of the benefits related to fasting. Recently, the role of fasting has shown promising results in promoting anti-cancer effects in the body.

Fasting reduces the ability of tumor cells to use glycolysis as a primary metabolic pathway for the breakdown of glucose and gain energy via a process known as the Warburg effect. Fasting helps in inducing oxidative phosphorylation in tumor cells that lead to increased oxidative stress and reduced levels of lactate and ATP in the cancer cell. As the ADP/ATP ratio is increased, it leads to the activation of the AMPK pathway, which promotes autophagy. Cell death occurs due to a constantly stressful environment. Fasting downregulates the MPAK pathway and suppresses the activation of AKT and mTOR pathways which induce autophagy that leads to the tumor cells' death. Furthermore, fasting also reduces chemotherapy-related damage to the DNA and helps in the early recovery of cells and organs.

Intermittent Fasting and Autophagy

It is not only important that we watch what we eat but also, when we eat.

What is Intermittent Fasting?

The physiology of the human body is quite interesting as it has its own biological clock according to which various processes occur daily. There is a 24-hour light/dark cycle which is controlled by natural circadian oscillators. These circadian oscillators are generally termed as a biological clock and have been conserved throughout the course of evolution. In this way, our body has its own time for various activities, such as being active, resting and regulating our intake of nutrients to ensure optimum function and longevity.

The idea of time-restricted feeding (tRF) has gained considerable attention in the past few years. Various studies in mice have shown that mice that undergo tRF consume the same number of calories in a high-fat diet as compared to the controls, but showed a decreased potential to develop obesity, hepatic steatosis, hyperinsulinemia, and inflammation. The physiological mechanism behind the protective effects of IF includes the regulation of AMPK, mTOR, and CREB pathways. These pathways also improve the cycles of the circadian clock and help in the optimum functioning of our biological clock. Studies suggest that fasting for five days can lead to a 30% decrease in glucose levels in the human body and around 50% decrease in the production of IGF-1, which is an important biomarker of aging and age-related diseases in humans.

Intermittent fasting is one type of time-restricted feeding which involves alternative cycles of eating and fasting. These cycles are comprised of 16 hours of fasting and 8 hours of mealtime, which can include 2 to 3 meals, in 24 hours. There are various types of intermittent fasting, such as the twice a week 16 hours fasting approach, alternate-day fasting, or a complete 24-hour fast once or twice a week. Most of the long-term fasting routines include an extended water fasting regime, which increases the benefits of fasting and promotes autophagy. In each type, intermittent fasting has fantastic benefits on the body.

There are five stages in intermittent fasting that start at 12 hours of fasting and end at 72 hours. Before going into the details of how intermittent fasting affects the body and what happens in each stage, it is necessary to understand what happens in the body when we are not fasting.

In a well-fed cell that has plenty of proteins and carbohydrates, the cell focuses only on dividing and growing. It wastes no time or energy on the cleanup or recycling process. During the growth phase, however, the genes of stress resistance, fat metabolism and damage repair are turned off, and the cell solely focuses on growth.

In the fasting state, the fat in the body is converted into ketone bodies that lead to the reactivation of these genes. These genes lead to the expression of proteins that are involved in the elimination of stress, as body senses starvation as a stress factor. The induced genes function to reduce inflammation, promote DNA repair and cause autophagic degradation of damaged and aged organelles and proteins. In this way, a complete set of proteins and biological processes that lead to the cleansing and replenishing of the cells and tissues are activated.

Fasting induces a self-preservation mode in the cell. It activates AMPK which promotes the breakdown of stored fat and induces autophagy. It also leads to the production of sirtuin proteins that are involved in the synthesis of new mitochondria and reduction of oxidative stress. The formation of ketone bodies during fasting also turn on genes related to damage repair and ant oxidation. All these beneficial processes occur in our body when we don't take in any calories and nutrients, ie., via the time-restricted feeding approach or intermittent fasting.

In the first stage of intermittent and prolonged fasting that is triggered by 12 hours of fasting, the process of ketosis is initiated. In this metabolic process, the body starts using fats as a source of energy. Ketone bodies are formed in the liver and utilized by the brain as an energy source in the absence of glucose. The utilization of ketone bodies by the brain cells help in the removal of inflammation and improve one's mood and mental clarity. By 24 hours of fasting, the cells in the brain and other tissues initiate the process of autophagy to recycle old components and degrade damaged proteins.

Autophagy promotes cellular rejuvenation and frees the cell from the burdens of damaged and inflamed proteins. Autophagy is directly linked with the process of aging, as the presence of inflamed and damaged organelles in the cell is considered as a hallmark of aging. Removal of these signs from the cell by autophagy highlights its importance. In this way, fasting improves the lifespan of an individual.

By 48 hours of low-calorie fasting, the production of various growth hormones is initiated. These hormones play an essential role in cardiovascular protection and in the healing of wounds and injured tissues. Prolonged fasting of 54 to 72 hours initiates the degradation of old immune cells and synthesizes new ones. Autophagy is the primary process that leads to the renewal and revamping of the immune system.

Protein Restriction

Proteins are necessary for the body but only in a limited amount. The importance of a well-balanced diet with respect to protein content is evident from the fact that young individuals who consume a high protein diet where they gain more than 20% of their caloric intake from protein, are more prone to various cancers and have shorter lifespans as compared to individuals who obtain less than 10% of their caloric intake from protein.

The amino acid deficiency during starvation leads to the induction of autophagy as autophagy is regulated by the perfect balance between fuel signaling pathways, mTOR and AMPK. These pathways can be considered as the yin and yang of the human metabolism. mTOR is the primary pathway that regulates the growth and induced anabolism and synthesis of protein. It is activated by the presence of amino acids, glucose and insulin, which leads to the inhibition of autophagy. In contrast to mTOR, the AMPK (AMP-Activated Protein Kinase) is a sensor of catabolism that promotes processes such as oxidation of fat and ketogenesis, and leads to the activation of autophagy.

AMPK is activated under energy-deprived conditions, protein restriction, exercise, and fasting.

Role of Various Dietary Components in Autophagy

As we already know that the availability of nutrients regulates the process of autophagy, there are certain dietary components that can directly regulate the level of autophagy. The major macronutrients, including fats, proteins and carbohydrates can mediate the autophagic rate and efficiency in the body. The building blocks of proteins and amino acids are one of the major regulators of autophagy. The presence of amino acids leads to the downregulation or inhibition of autophagy, while the absence of amino acids during the starvation phase leads to the induction of autophagy. Among the different amino acids, the most efficient mediators of autophagy include phenylalanine, leucine and tyrosine. The mTOR pathway mediates the amino acid-based suppression of autophagy as amino acids can increase the intracellular levels of calcium which lead to the activation of the mTOR Complex 1. This complex, when activated, acts as a suppressor of autophagy. The levels of amino acids change according to our diet and intake of proper protein can help regulate the level of autophagy in the cells and body.

Lipids and carbohydrates play an indirect role in the regulation of autophagy. The primary effector of carbohydrates is insulin and levels of this hormone directly mediate the process of autophagy. The catabolism of carbohydrates leads to the release of glucose which is the primary energy source of the cells. Glucose plays an important role in the regulation of endocrine pathways including the insulin pathway. Increased cellular levels of glucose and insulin lead to the activation of the mTOR pathway, which means autophagy is inhibited. Also, the increase in glucose leads to increased levels of NADH through glycolysis which suppresses the activity of sirtuin, another regulator of autophagy. The decreased activity of sirtuin leads to the suppression of autophagy. The presence of high levels of glucose in the cell means that the cell is well fed and the nutrient recycling process, ie., autophagy, is rendered inactive.

The role of fats in the induction of autophagy is quite interesting as high levels of fatty acids in serum develop insulin resistance in the cell. This leads to the inactivation of mTOR which encourages the cell to activate autophagy.

Anti-aging Pharmacological Mimetics for Inducing Autophagy

The challenge of adhering to prolonged CR regimes has led to the development of much safer and convenient alternatives to calorie restriction to achieve autophagy and its anti-aging benefits. Also, there are certain side effects of practicing prolonged CR, which include a delay in healing of wounds and a decrease in body temperature. The search for a pharmacological answer to this has led to the use of various calorie restriction mimetic (CRM) supplements to delay the aging process primarily by the induction of autophagy. The most widely studied and used CRM supplements are spermidine, resveratrol, rapamycin and metformin.

Spermidine

Spermidine is a polyamine that is naturally produced by the body. It is known to play an important role in the determination of lifespan by inducing autophagy. As we age, there is a gradual decline in the production of spermidine. It has been reported that in humans, the use of spermidine dietary supplementation for two months leads to an increase in the blood polyamine concentrations. Spermidine is a non-toxic compound and its use for humans is completely safe. The autophagy-inducing potential of spermidine has been found to be equivalent to rapamycin.

Studies show that the loss of autophagic activity due to the suppression of Atg7 leads to a decrease in lifespan and loss of neuroprotection *in vivo*. In recent decades, the use of spermidine-based dietary supplements has shown promising results in preventing aging and has reduced the risk of Alzheimer's disease. There is experimental evidence that the use of nutritional spermidine leads to delay in age-related memory loss. However, the exact dose for enabling healthy aging by inducing optimal autophagy using spermidine supplements in humans remains unknown.

Resveratrol

Resveratrol is a polyphenol compound. It is naturally obtained from red grapes and blueberry peels. The dietary intake of polyphenols from fruits has gained interest as a preferable source of autophagy induction through calorie restriction effects. Resveratrol is considered as the most potent polyphenol compound. The use of resveratrol has shown positive effects in the treatment and prevention of neurodegenerative diseases. It has been proved to be beneficial for improving age-related cognitive disabilities and has implications in extending the lifespan in yeast models.

There are various physiological effects of resveratrol in the body which mediate its anti-aging and neuroprotective action. Resveratrol causes an increase in the insulin sensitivity, a reduction in IGF1 levels, and activates the AMPK/PGC-1α signaling pathway. It also plays an important role in improving the motor functions of the nervous system. Resveratrol causes a reduction in the inflammatory response caused by the intake of a fat-rich diet and prevents the diet-induced inflammation of the arterial wall.

Despite of having so many benefits for the human body, naturally-occurring resveratrol is poorly absorbed and metabolized by the humans. Hence, various highly effective resveratrol-mimetic drugs, have been developed, for instance, ResVida™. It has been found that the use of resveratrol supplements for one month can lead to a decrease in the levels of circulating glucose, triglycerides, inflammatory markers, and systolic blood pressure. The long-term use of resveratrol supplements has been considered safe for humans.

Longevinex® is another resveratrol supplement that is used commercially. It can induce SIRT1 and has been linked with an increase in levels of Beclin1, LC3-II and FOXO transcription factors. These effects suggest that Longevinex® has beneficial effects on the brain as it increases the rate of mitochondrial biogenesis in the brain and induces neuronal autophagy. Resveratrol can induce the AMPK pathway in the brain cells and can rid the cells from the accumulation of extracellular Aβ by inducing autophagy. Various studies in mice have shown that long term use of resveratrol led to improved memory and reduced the level of Aβ in the brain tissues, which makes it a promising candidate for the treatment of Alzheimer's disease.

Rapamycin

Rapamycin is one of the most widely studied and used autophagy inducers. It is a major suppressor of mTORC1 activity which has been associated to have significant benefits for both health and lifespan in various organisms. It is also one of the most widely used supplements for calorie restriction mimetics. Rapamycin is FDA-approved and can be used for various clinical applications in humans.

Various studies on neurodegenerative disorders using mouse models show that the treatment of affected cells with rapamycin led to an improvement in cognitive ability and reduction in Aβ aggregates. The underlying mechanism of action has been found to be the induction of autophagy, which functions to degrade and remove the aggregates and clears the signs of aging and disease from brain cells. Prolonged use of rapamycin has been found to be associated with expansion of lifespan in mice.

Rapatar is a commercially available formulation of rapamycin. It has a significantly higher bioavailability as compared to naturally-occurring rapamycin. Rapatar has been proven to be beneficial in increasing the lifespan and delaying tumor progression upon lifelong treatment in mice.

Metformin

Metformin is a known drug that is used for the treatment of diabetes. It regulates the blood glucose and insulin levels by targeting various pathways, including the AMPK pathway, mTORC1, insulin/IGF1 pathway, and SIRT1. The regulation of these pathways, which regulate the process of autophagy, makes metformin an important candidate for regulating autophagy in the body. Some of the major metabolic effects of metformin that links its association with autophagy include neuroprotective effects as it lowers the risk of AD in diabetic patients by inducing neuronal autophagy and the removal of Aβ oligomers from brain tissue.

Food that Promotes Autophagy

As autophagy is primarily regulated by the nutrient status of the body, various nutrients and dietary components play an important in the upregulation of autophagy.

Our diet and nutrient intake play an essential role in our body and have far more complex impacts on our body than simply providing energy. The intake of the right nutrients and using food as medicine can have extraordinary effects on our body and its metabolism. Autophagy is a natural process, yet certain foods and nutrients can help in triggering autophagy in our body. Some of these autophagy-promoting foods are given below:

- Consumption of dark-green, leafy vegetables, including kale, spinach, etc., can help in the induction of autophagy in the body. These vegetables are rich in sulforaphane that promote autophagy through the activation of extracellular signal-regulated kinase (ERK) in the nerve cell. Similarly, polyphenols that are also present in green, leafy vegetables and cherries help in promoting autophagy.

- Certain mushrooms, such as the chaga mushroom and various other species are helpful in inducing autophagy in the body.

- Consumption of ginger is advised for the triggering of autophagy as it contains a compound known as 6-

shogaol, which induces autophagy through the inhibition of AKT/mTOR pathway in the cells. Turmeric, which contains curcumin, can also induce autophagy through the activation of the AMPK pathway.

- Consuming a considerable amount of coffee is recommended for the induction of autophagy and is part of various diets that are designed to promote autophagy, such as the keto diet. Coffee promotes ketosis, regulates blood sugar, and has a high content of polyphenol, which makes it a perfect triggering factor for autophagy.

- Green tea can trigger autophagy as it is rich in polyphenols. It causes induction of autophagy, especially in liver cells.

- Certain fruits, such as berries, cherries and dark grapes, are recommended to induce autophagy in the body. These fruits contain resveratrol that promotes autophagy.

- Consumption of olive oil (extra virgin) is highly recommended for the induction of autophagy. It contains various polyphenols such as oleuropein and oleocanthal, which trigger autophagy through the suppression of mTOR.

- Various foods such as salmon, algae, mackerel and flax seeds are also considered as important sources of autophagy inducers. These contain omega-3 polyunsaturated fatty acids that induce autophagy.

- Similarly, eggs, liver, pumpkin seeds and red meat are also beneficial in the triggering of autophagy. The presence of a high amount of zinc acts as an essential inducer of autophagy in the body.

Autophagy-Inducing Foods

There are certain foods and food components that are widely researched for therapeutic purposes due to their autophagy-inducing abilities. These dietary components provide a natural means for the treatment of various diseases, including neurodegenerative diseases, metabolic disorders, and cancers. The mechanism of action of these foods is primarily the induction of autophagy. However, there are various direct and indirect cellular pathways of autophagy that are influenced by the active components of the food. Some of the most widely studied and most effective food and food components that can lead to the induction of autophagy in the cells are given below:

Caffeine

Caffeine is the major active component of cocoa, tea and coffee. It is also added to colas and drinks as a flavoring agent. Caffeine can induce autophagy in the body. Various studies suggest that treatment of microbial cells with a small concentration of caffeine can lead to induction of autophagy. In humans, caffeine acts an inducer of autophagy as it inhibits the production of various kinase enzymes that are part of mTOR pathway. Caffeine also plays various roles in other vital processes of the cells, including apoptosis, and affects cell cycle regulatory proteins such as p53. Caffeine also has positive effects on the health of our brain and neurological system. It can improve our cognitive abilities and has been shown to help patients with neurodegenerative diseases, such as Parkinson's, in managing their symptoms. It is assumed that these neuroprotective effects of caffeine are attributed to the induction of autophagy in brain cells. Consumption of coffee and other caffeine-containing products have been linked with an increase in lifespan, a trait that is also attributed to autophagy.

Curcumin

Curcumin is a natural compound that is present in turmeric. It is the active component of turmeric which gives the yellow color to curry and has a distinct taste. Curcumin is a biologically active compound and has been used in various therapeutic medicines, including anticancer drugs. The mechanism of action of curcumin involves its vital role in the production of the autophagosome, and thereby, autophagy. It induces cell death in abnormal cells through the activation of autophagy. Treatment of various cancerous cell lines with a controlled amount of curcumin has been shown to cause an increase in the production of autophagic vesicles and autophagosomes in cells. This increase leads to the destruction and death of the cancerous cells and thus depicts the anti-cancer potential of turmeric. A daily dose of up to 100 mg/day can be ingested from food and is considered nontoxic. The bioavailability of ingested curcumin is quite low but can be enhanced by ingesting pepper with curcumin, which contains piperine.

Curcumin has been a part of traditional medicine since early times. The use of turmeric has been beneficial for curing various inflammatory and neurodegenerative diseases, primarily due to its autophagic potential.

Fenugreek

Fenugreek is a leguminous plant, native to countries in Asia and the Middle East. It is used in various forms, including whole-seed and ground-state as a source of protein. The active component of fenugreek has been shown to induce vacuolization in various tissues which suggests its autophagic role. Various studies suggest that fenugreek extracts have protective effects against cancer as cells exposed to cancer-inducing compounds failed to affect the fenugreek-treated cells as compared to untreated cells. The treated cells showed an increased amount of autophagosomes that contained damaged organelles and other cytoplasmic materials and hence protected the cell through autophagy.

Vitamin C

Vitamin C is found in many vegetables and fruits and is most prevalent in citrus fruits. It is also known as ascorbic acid and it provides amazing health benefits. Vitamin C has anti-cancer properties and studies suggest that the treatment of cancer cells with vitamin C induces the production of autophagic vesicles and leads to the removal of damaged organelles and cells. Similarly, patients with neurodegenerative diseases have a low level of vitamin C in the serum, which suggests a low level of autophagy that can cause problems with the neuronal system and neurodegeneration. A daily intake of around five fruits and vegetables is equivalent to 250 mg of vitamin C, which is enough to meet the bioavailability of vitamin C in the body and meet our body's needs.

Vitamin D

One of the most important and prevalent components of our diet is calcium and vitamin D. Various analogs and supplements of calcium and vitamin D are used along with natural sources such as fish, dairy products and the sun to fulfill the nutrient requirements of our body. The effect of vitamin D on various human tissues shows that there was an increase in the production of autophagosomes and the process of autophagy. Vitamin D mediates the levels of calcium in the body, which influences the mTOR pathway. The inhibition of mTOR leads to the induction of the autophagic process. Various studies show the protective role of vitamin D against breast, ovarian and colon cancer. The primary mechanism of action through which vitamin D confers anti-cancer effects is through autophagic destruction and death of cancerous cells.

Sulphoraphane

Sulphoraphane is a potent anti-cancer compound found in various plants, including cruciferous vegetables. This compound affects various vital processes in the cell, including the cell cycle, apoptosis, protection from genotoxic damage and autophagy. Sulphoraphane has shown positive effects on cancerous cells from prostate tissues, where treatment with this compound led to an increase in the autophagic structures in the cells. The cytoprotective effects of autophagy were found to be associated with a decline in the release of cytochrome, which helps in the destruction of cancerous cells. Sulphoraphane also affects the expression of Bcl-2; decrease in Bcl-2 leads to the activation of Beclin-1. And as described above, Beclin-1 plays an important role in the activation of autophagy.

Tocotrienols

These compounds are derivates of vitamin E and are naturally present in rice bran and palm oil. They have neuroprotective and anti-tumor properties and various studies suggest that these health-promoting effects of tocotrienols are attributed to their ability to induce autophagy in the cells.

Lithium

Lithium belongs to a group of alkali metals in the periodic table. It is naturally present in meat, grains, vegetables, and water. Animal studies show that the treatment of kidney cells with lithium causes an increase in the number of autophagosomes. This autophagic effect was elicited through the inhibition of inositol monophosphate rather than the mTOR signaling pathway. The autophagy-inducing ability of lithium has been linked with its role in protection against Huntington disease, which is a neurodegenerative disorder that is characterized by the formation and accumulation of huntingtin protein aggregates in the body. Moreover, the role of lithium in the induction of autophagy can be exploited for the degradation and removal of mutant α-synuclein protein aggregates, which cause Parkinson's disease.

Luteolin

Luteolin is a naturally occurring flavone. It is found in celery, chamomile tea, green pepper and perilla seeds. It has been identified as a down regulator of the autophagic process. Luteolin has anti-tumorigenic properties and has shown positive results in the treatment of oral squamous cell carcinoma. Luteolin inhibits autophagy, which helps the survival and progression of cancer cells as they avoid apoptosis. Therefore, by reducing autophagy, we can induce apoptosis or cell death of cancer cells which can aid in anti-cancer therapy.

MK615

MK615 is a natural compound. It is obtained from Japanese apricot and has anticancer properties. MK615 can inhibit the proliferation of breast cancer cells and induce apoptosis in them, leading to cell death. Furthermore, upon treatment with MK615, there was an increase in the number of autophagic vesicles in the cancerous cells. Similar findings have been reported from studies on colon cancer cells which highlight the ant proliferative and apoptosis-inducing effects of MK615, which are attributed to autophagy.

Apigenin

A major regulator of autophagy that is found in a wide range of herbs and plants is apigenin. It is present in pepper, oregano, thyme, parsley, rosemary, olives, and celery.

Benzyl Isothiocyanate

Benzyl isothiocyanate is primarily present in cruciferous vegetables. It has been known to have chemoprotective properties. Treatment of breast cancer cells with a controlled amount of benzyl isothiocyanate led to cell cycle arrest, apoptosis, and an increase in the production of autophagosomes.

Bromovanin

Bromovanin is present in vanillin and gives the distinct flavor and aroma of vanilla. Various studies suggest that the treatment of various cells with bromovanin led to an increase in the production of the autophagosome, thus marking the induction of autophagy. Bromovanin can also induce apoptosis, decrease the activity of certain kinases, and increase the production of ROS (reactive oxygen species), which also promote autophagy.

Triterpenoid Saponins (Group B)

These compounds are present primarily in soya products and are termed as soyasaponins. They are a subclass of triterpenoids which have various health benefits. Triterpenoids are predominant in intact legumes and have been investigated for their effects on autophagy. Soy products contain B-group triterpenoids, which includes saponins and genistein. They have anti-cancer properties. High amount of soy products in the diet have been linked with decreased levels of prostate and breast cancer, and these anti-cancer effects have been linked to an increase in the production of autophagic vesicles upon treatment with saponins and genistein.

Autophagy and Weight Loss

The importance of autophagy and autophagy-inducing factors in controlling the weight of the body has been highlighted in recent years. Autophagy is a catabolic process that influences the nutrient status of the body. Furthermore, it also mediates the process of fat metabolism and glucose levels in the body. Various studies in mice models show that induction of autophagy through calorie restriction led to weight loss in healthy mice as compared to the experimental mice which lack the autophagy gene *atg4b*. These findings suggest that there is a definitive role of autophagy in controlling body mass and weight. The systemic activity of autophagy provides protection forth organism against gain weight when subjected to a diet that is rich in calories.

Exercise, Training, and Autophagy

Physical activity increases strength, endurance and makes our metabolism top notch

The Difference between Exercise and Training

Exercise and training refers to both physical activity and workouts. However, there is a certain technical difference between the two as exercise is performed to get immediate effects from a workout, such as burning calories, building biceps, stretching, and shedding some sweat, whereas training is a physical activity that is designed and performed to achieve a goal and is about the process of learning something through specific physical exercise and endurance activities.

In both forms, physical activity is considered as an important factor for the health and wellbeing of the body. And one of the most vital roles of exercise in the body is that it acts as a trigger for autophagy.

Benefits of Exercise In Relation to Autophagy

Exercise causes a sharp increase in the consumption of oxygen and energy that results in the decrease of nutrients and oxygen, and an increase in oxidative stress by the generation of reactive oxygen species (ROS). These cellular conditions act as a trigger for the process of autophagy that aids the cell in coping with a stressful environment.

Exercise-induced autophagy has been observed in various tissues and organs of the body. For instance, the liver, adipose tissues, skeletal muscle, pancreas, cardiac muscle, and cerebral cortex are some of the most significant issues that undergo exercise-induced autophagy. Physical exercise has many beneficial effects on our health, which includes an increase the in life-span, and protects the body from diabetes, neurodegenerative disorders and various types of cancers — most of the health benefits of exercise overlap with known protective roles of autophagy.

Various studies suggest that exercise and training can increase the rate of autophagy to maintain the physiological activities of skeletal muscle. Other benefits of exercise that primarily affect the health of cardiac tissues involve the inhibition of apoptosis that has occurred due to myocardial infarction, reduction in myocardial cell damage and improvement of cardiovascular function. Aerobic exercise induces autophagy that protects cardiac cells.

Proper exercise and training at a favorable intensity can induce autophagy that helps in the degradation and removal of metabolic waste that is necessary to maintain the steady-state of the cell.

Improving Energy Metabolism

Exercise and training play an important role in enhancing the metabolic system and efficiency in the body. It does so by affecting the turnover rate of mitochondria. This means that it improves the synthesis of mitochondria and induces autophagy to remove the aged or damaged mitochondria from the cell. In this way, exercise ensures that enough healthy mitochondria that function at their best and maintain the proficiency of metabolism are present.

Moreover, autophagy and microRNA-mediated autophagy are involved in the regulation of the removal of unwanted organelles from the cell and promote the adaptation of muscles and metabolism towards exercise.

Various studies have researched the role of exercise in the induction of autophagy in multiple tissues and parts of the body. Some of the most significant tissues where exercise-related autophagy is triggered are skeletal muscles which are discussed below.

Autophagy in Skeletal Muscles

The role of exercise training in mediating the process of autophagy has become a hot spot in the field of exercise science. In 1984, it was reported that endurance exercise and high-intensity workouts promote the induction of autophagy in skeletal muscle. Experiments on mice that were subjected to high-intensity treadmill training showed that the strongest autophagy response was observed within 48 hours after exercise.

Exercise and training accelerate the metabolic processes involving the catabolism and anabolism of fatty acids, proteins, and, glucose. It also promotes the biogenesis of mitochondria, influences the process of angiogenesis, and causes a delay in the aging of skeletal muscle. All these effects are attributed to the process of autophagy that is induced by exercise training.

High-altitude training leads to the induction of the process of autophagy which eventually improves exercise performance. High-altitude training induces autophagy and mitophagy that aids in the maintenance of the quality of skeletal muscle by eliminating abnormal and aged mitochondria from the cell. This cleansing process promotes the efficiency of energy metabolism that is required by the cell to fulfill the increased energy needs.

High altitude training also leads to the activation of HIF-1 that stimulates the expression of vascular endothelial factor (VEGF) and erythropoietin (EPO). These growth factors increase the mass of hemoglobin and the density of capillaries in the muscle.

Autophagy prepares the body and strengthens the metabolic process of the cell to endure exercise and high-altitude training. Aerobic and hypoxic training exercises lead to the induction of autophagy, which suggests that autophagy is the molecular mechanism of the adaptive response of the body to exercise and high-altitude training. The production of autophagic biomarkers during endurance exercises and high-altitude training might provide useful insight into the potential of an individual for such training. However, extreme exercise and training can cause excessive autophagy that can lead to excessive degradation of protein and loss of skeletal muscle.

Thus, we can say that autophagy in skeletal muscle plays a significant role in maintaining its quality and structure. The regulation of protein degradation as well synthesis of proteins by autophagy is equally vital for ensuring the health of skeletal muscles after endurance exercise and training.

Mechanism of autophagy in Skeletal Muscles

Various changes in the biochemistry of autophagy in the skeletal muscles help the muscles adapt to its changing energy needs. When muscles are subjected to bouts of high-intensity exercise, it leads to the induction of autophagy in both oxidative and glycolytic muscles. It also leads to a reduction in the synthesis of proteins during the exercise period and an increase in protein synthesis later in the recovery period. For young adults, the use of acute-endurance training proves to be more beneficial, while the use of resistance-training in older age can have similar benefits on the body as both induce autophagy and help in improving the strength and endurance of the muscles.

Doing an Autophagy Session

Autophagy can be induced through the right diet and exercise, so it is highly recommended that we treat ourselves with the extraordinary benefits of autophagy. It is a natural detox process for our body and helps us achieve the desirable concept of *healthy aging*!

After reading the above section, we can pick some quick and easy tips that will help in the induction of autophagy in our body:

1. Practice a high-intensity training session that is comprised of sprints and strength training as this will trigger autophagy.

2. To increase autophagy, fasting for two or three days a week is highly recommended.

3. It is very beneficial to stay active and on our feet throughout our fast. This will help ramp up the metabolism of fats and lead to ketosis, which further induces autophagy in our cells.

4. During intermittent fasting, drink as much coffee as possible as it is a strong inducer of autophagy.

5. Follow a high-fat, low-carbohydrate diet plan and limit your protein intake. This diet plan will boost the process of autophagy.

6. Get proper sleep so that your body can rest and recover through autophagy.

Autophagy Inducing Supplements and Therapies

Apart from diet and exercise, there are certain supplements and therapies that are used at the clinical level to induce autophagy. Such clinical approaches have gained worldwide attention as autophagy acts as a natural cleanser of the body and hence has a significant role in the elimination and treatment of various ailments and diseases. Moreover, multiple supplements and compounds have been developed that artificially induce autophagy in the body. This is a novel approach to autophagy regulation as most of these supplements do not require mTOR for the induction of the autophagic process and can independently regulate it.

Some of the few FDA approved compounds that are used for promoting autophagy in humans are given in **Table 4.**

Table 4. The list of compounds that have the potential to induce autophagy

Sr #	Compounds	Autophagy Induction Mechanism
1	Carbamazepine	Decreases the level of inositol in the body
2	Sodium valproate	Decreases the level of inositol in the body
3	Metformin	Decreases the level of AMPK and induces beclin1 and ULK1
4	Verapamil	Decreases the level of intra-cytosolic calcium
5	Clonidine	Decreases the level of cAMP in the cells
6	Tyrosine kinase inhibitors	Induces the level of beclin1 and inhibits mTOR
7	Trifluoperazine	Mechanism not known
8	Rilmenidine	Decreases the level of cAMP in the cells
9	Rapamycin	Inhibits the production of mTORC1
10	Statins	Activates the production of AMPK
11	Lithium	Decreases the level of inositol in the body

There are some nutritional supplements that are recommended by physicians to promote the process of autophagy (**Table 5**).

Table 5. List of dietary supplements that have the potential to induce autophagy

Sr #	Compounds	**Autophagy Induction Mechanism**
1	Vitamin D	Induces transcriptional genes through calcium signaling
2	Resveratrol	Induces sirtuin 1
3	Caffeine	Suppresses mTOR signaling
4	Spermidine	Inhibits acetylase
5	Trehalose	Not known
6	Omega-3 polyunsaturated fatty acid	Inhibits the signaling of m-TOR

Clinical Approaches to Induce Autophagy

Various clinical approaches are used to regulate and induce autophagy in the body. Three of the most common therapeutic methods related to autophagy are given below:

- Autophagy gene therapy
- Transgenic expression of autophagy
- Autophagy-inducing peptides

The systemic expression of the autophagy-related gene Atg5 has been shown to induce positive effects in mice models. It has led to the expansion of the lifespan, and an end-efficient metabolism profile.

Various autophagy-related genes are being used as targets to improve various clinical conditions. Gene therapy involves the tissue-specific delivery of autophagic genes using different vectors or carriers. Through this method, the most important autophagy-related genes, including Atg7, Beclin-1 and Tfeb have been delivered to liver, brain, and muscle cells to aid in the treatment of various liver and muscular disorders.

Autophagy-related gene therapies have shown an improvement in the function of hepatic insulin and systemic glucose tolerance in mice. They have also shown positive results in the treatment of lysosomal storage muscle disease in muscles, such as Pompe disease. Gene therapy using autophagy-related genes have great potential in treating neurodegenerative diseases, such as Parkinson's and Alzheimer's disease.

Various autophagy-inducing peptides, including Tat-Beclin-1, have been shown to have therapeutic potential as this peptide is designed to induce autophagy in multiple diseased cells and tissues.

Screening for Autophagy-Inducing CRMs

Among various nutritional and chemical supplements that are used to induce autophagy in the body, the use of autophagy-inducing drugs for the attenuation of risks that are associated with different age-associated diseases is becoming common. Recently, an autophagic flux probe has been developed. This probe can analyze and rank different autophagy-inducing drugs based on their potency level by screening through a known drug library. The autophagic flux probe is GFP-LC3-RFP-LC3ΔG. It is a fusion protein and gives out a signal when autophagy occurs in the body; this signal is then analyzed against a candidate drug that is being screened for its autophagy-inducing potential. A low GFP/RFP ratio indicates a strong autophagy inducer. By using this approach, various autophagy inducers have been identified. They are specified in Table 6 along with the pathologies for which the drugs have been proved to be beneficial by inducing autophagy.

Table 6. The list of useful drugs for the induction of autophagy identified via probe method

Serial #	Drug	Disease	GFP/RFP (%)
1	Ciclopirox olamine	Cancer	1
2	Cladribine	Alzheimer's	51.1

	(2-CDA)	Disease	
3	Sertraline hydrochloride	Depression	58.8
4	Loperamide hydrochloride	Hematopoiesis disorders	70
5	Azacytidine	Huntington Disease	61.7

Various antiaging nutrients that induce autophagy have been identified using this probe. These nutrients include antioxidants, which include vitamins A, D, and E and related coenzymes, as well as various phytochemicals including curcumin.

The Ideal Diet for Successful Aging

Nutrition transition and preferable dietary patterns have evolved around the world and different regions and cultures have unique eating habits. It has been found that regions including Asia, Middle East, Latin America and sub-Saharan African countries have relatively similar dietary patterns. Various studies on age-associated diseases and dietary patterns have highlighted the role of nutrients and food with the increased risk of age-associated diseases in this region. This region has become bound to the consumption of high fat and high sugar foods, and this commonality is proportional to the ratio of age-associated diseases in the people of these regions.

On the other hand, in regions where the Okinawan diet is common, people are less prone to age-related disorders. This diet includes low-GI grains, sweet potatoes, leguminous plants, carotenoid-rich food and different kinds of flavonoids. Such a dietary regime is considered as part of calorie restriction (CR) practices and has been considered to be the most advantageous dietary choice for successful aging. The underlying process behind the benefits of such a calorie-restricted diet has been found to be autophagy, which cleanses the body and plays an important role in achieving longevity.

Sleep as a Regulator of Autophagy

Sleep better and recover faster through autophagy

Sleep is considered a necessary and effective treatment of various conditions as it is the time when our body rests and heals itself. The sleep and wake cycle are an essential part of the circadian rhythm, or the internal biological clock of the body. The natural clock of our body regulates all the vital processes in our body. Autophagy is among one of them.

The activation of autophagy in cells is well controlled and follows a rhythmic cycle. The natural biological clock works according to the division of day and night, or a cycle of sleep and wakefulness. Sleep acts as an essential regulator of autophagy and disruption of sleep cycles. A lack of sleep can affect the functionality of the circadian rhythm and can compromise the accuracy and efficiency of autophagy.

There is a close coupling between the biological clock and the autophagic degradation process that maintains energy homeostasis in the body. This coupling also helps in the remodeling of cell organelles and proteins, compartmentalization of tissue metabolism, and provides a balance of nutrients. The circadian autophagy is regulated by two cues, the time of day and nutritional signals. So, if we follow the natural sleep and wakefulness cycle as determined by our biological clock, the process of the circadian rhythm of autophagy also works in an optimum manner to regulate vital metabolic processes.

Getting good quality sleep has been linked with a healthy body and mind whereas sleep deprivation is associated with various neurological and physiological disorders and a decrease in lifespan. The importance of sleep is due to the different essential processes that occur during sleeping, and a lack of sleep causes disruption of these vital physiological processes.

The vital processes that occur during sleep include the physical repair of muscles and organs, muscle growth, consolidation of memory, loss of fat and autophagy. Moreover, sleep is vital for brain functions as various toxic proteins and beta-amyloid are cleared from the brain through autophagy. This autophagic removal of beta-amyloid is crucial in the protection from Alzheimer's disease.

Moreover, autophagy is regulated by certain hormones. Melatonin, that is a sleep hormone that greatly influences autophagy. It prepares the body for beneficial processes such as growth and repair through autophagy. Autophagy also occurs in during the diurnal rhythm in heart, muscles, and liver in mice and has an increased rate at periods of low metabolic activity such as sleep. Furthermore, nearly all metabolic processes including the biosynthesis of cholesterol, beta-oxidation of fatty acids and gluconeogenesis in the liver, occur at rhythmical cycles and autophagy is involved in these processes to ensure nutrient supply for oxidation as well as storage. Thus, autophagy is intensely regulated by the biological clock and our sleep-wakefulness cycles. Ensuring proper and deep sleep helps our body to cleanse and repair itself through autophagy.

The recommended amount of sleep varies from 6 to 8 hours; however, time and quality of sleep are more significant than the number of sleeping hours. A few hours of sound sleep at night is more beneficial than sleeping for long hours during the daytime. Following the sleep cycle as determined by our biological clock and maintaining the circadian rhythms of the body will upregulate the process of autophagy and improve our health and lifespan. A lack of sleep causes the internal clock to become out of sync with the environment and can lead to stress and inflammation in the body.

AUTOPHAGY AND OBESITY

Autophagy is a degradative process. It plays an important role in managing various stresses in the body, including obesity and related stresses. These stresses include oxidative stresses, proteotoxic stress, and obesity-associated toxicity. Obesity is a global problem that affects around 2.1 billion people, approximately 30% of the population. Autophagy helps in maintaining the homeostasis of the body by coping with the stresses related to obesity. However, obesity can compromise or inhibit the process of autophagy at various levels. This can lead to worsening of obesity-related metabolic pathologies that can cause dysfunction in multiple organs.

On the other hand, there are certain studies that suggest that the inhibition of autophagy under certain conditions can have beneficial effects in reducing various damaging consequences of obesity. So, autophagy plays a dual role in obesity and related pathologies. It can protect as well as promote the damages of obesity under different conditions. This role of autophagy highlights its importance in the metabolic and physiological pathways of the body, as obesity is a multifactorial disease and results in pathologies that may affect various organs of the body. For instance, obesity is commonly associated with diverse comorbidities, including cardiovascular disease, hypertension, diabetes, dyslipidemia and cancer. The autophagic catabolism plays a significant role in preventing the complications of obesity and a lack of autophagy can have deleterious effects on the health, especially in obese individuals.

Stresses Related to Obesity

The major cause of obesity is our modern lifestyle, which primarily entails a lack of physical activity, an unhealthy diet, and over-nutrition. This has led to the current epidemic of obesity and it is getting worse with every passing day. Obesity results from the consumption of surplus calories that get stored as fat in the adipose tissue. The accumulation of fat can also occur in non-adipose tissue, including the skeletal muscles and liver, which can be damaging to these tissues. Moreover, the accumulation of excessive fat can increase the level of free fatty acids in the serum which is characterized as systemic lipotoxicity.

All biological membranes have lipids as an integral part of their system. The presence of excessive influx and accumulation of lipids can affect cellular function by altering the fluidity and integrity of their membranes. Obesity can lead to changes in the lipidomic profile of various organelles, including the endoplasmic reticulum (ER). This can compromise the process of protein synthesis and lead to the accumulation of unfolded proteins. These unfolded proteins have toxic effects on the ER which leads to lipogenesis. The proteotoxic effects can also trigger various lipotoxic pathologies. Presence of high level of lipids can induce various stress responses, including oxidative stress by the production of ROS, the stress of signaling pathway, and stress-activated protein kinase signaling that triggers obesity-related metabolic pathologies. The metabolites of fatty acids can indirectly activate stress signaling pathways in the cell. Together, these responses lead to a magnification of pathologies or complications of obesity, such as insulin resistance and chronic inflammation.

Autophagy is a major stress-combating process of the body and helps the cells in maintaining their function by fighting off various stresses. Autophagy plays a protective role against the lipid-induced stresses in the following ways:

- Autophagy eliminates and destroys the lipid droplets through the process called lipophagy. This reduces the fat content and normalizes the metabolism of lipids in the tissues of obese individuals.

- Autophagy eliminates dysfunctional mitochondria through a process called mitophagy. This reduces the production of ROS and protects the cells from obesity-associated pathologies and DNA damage.

- During ER stress, autophagy can fight ER stress by eliminating a part of the ER through a process called ER-phagy. This removes the damaged parts of the ER and restores its homeostasis.

In this way, autophagy plays a very crucial role in the resolution of obesity-associated stresses in the body and provides protection against the clinical complications of obesity. However, it has been reported that obesity and obesity-related stresses can interfere with the process of autophagy and make it ineffective. The absence of autophagy in the cells can make them vulnerable to the damages of obesity. There are various ways through which obesity and related stresses can compromise autophagic process. They will be discussed in the next section.

Effects of Obesity on Autophagy

Initially, it was believed that the process of autophagy is inactive during obesity. In conditions of hyper-nutrition when the cell is well fed, the autophagy process is turned off by the inhibition of AMPK and activation of mTORC1. Various studies suggest that the activity of mTORC1 is triggered during obesity and is linked with an increase in the synthesis of energy reserves in the liver. Many studies that involved obese mice show that there is a downregulation of the autophagic process in test subjects. Genetic analysis shows a reduction in expression of the ATG5 and ATG7 genes that indicate a decrease in the production of the autophagosome. The comorbidities of obesity, insulin resistance and hyper-insulinemia also have inhibitory effects on the process of autophagy during obesity. The lipotoxic stress can decrease the AMPK signaling which can decrease the production of the autophagosome in various cells, including liver cells and macrophages.

All these studies suggest that the process of autophagy is downregulated by obesity and its related stresses. However, recent studies in human and mouse tissues show that there is an increase in the production of autophagosomes in response to obesity and related lipotoxic stress in various tissues, including adipose and liver tissues. These findings show that the connection between autophagy and obesity is not as simple as was speculated originally, and that autophagy plays a more crucial role in obesity and related pathologies.

There is more evidence that autophagy process is upregulated in obesity. It has been reported that ER stress—the hallmark of obesity and lipotoxicity—can cause the induction of autophagy via several mechanisms. Obesity itself is a strong inducer of ER stress in the liver cells. Obesity-associated ER stress increases the accumulation of fat in various tissues and cause insulin resistance and damage to liver cells. In this way, autophagy is induced by obesity and related stresses as a defensive mechanism to protect cells from the damages of ER stress.

In fibroblasts, protein kinase C (PKC) is activated by the lipotoxic effects on the cell. The activation of this protein upregulates the autophagic flux which protects the cell from apoptosis. Other stresses linked to obesity include oxidative stress and inflammation and have also been reported as strong inducers of autophagy. These stresses can upregulate autophagy via multiple pathways. In obesity-related stress, the induction of autophagy can be characterized as a cellular defense mechanism. It ensures cell survival by maintaining the cellular homeostasis in unfavorable stress conditions.

However, the induction of autophagy in lipid-overloaded cells should result in a decrease in the accumulation of lipid droplets. However, the findings show the opposite reaction. The autophagic process fails to decrease this accumulation and there is an increase in substrate levels in various cells due to obesity and lipotoxicity. These findings propose that obesity can interfere with the efficiency of autophagy.

Studies have shown that there is an increase in the production of autophagosomes in cells of obese individuals, but the actual parameter that determines the efficiency of autophagy process, the autophagic flux, is reduced. So, the upregulation of autophagy as evident by the production of vesicles can be seen in obesity and associated stresses, but the process is not carried out in the way it should be. There is a certain kind of interference from the obesity-associated stresses that lead to a fizzled autophagic process.

This defect in the degradative abilities of autophagy is of the leading causes of the accumulation of autophagosomes during obesity. Such accumulation has been reported in pancreatic beta cells, as well as liver and kidney cells from obese individuals. The inhibition of catabolic action of autophagy in obese individuals is carried out by various mechanisms.

It has been reported that lipotoxic stress can interfere with the autophagic flux through different mechanisms in different tissues. Thus, this inhibition of autophagic flux is a tissue-dependent mechanism and varies according to the tissues in which autophagy have been induced under obesity-related stresses.

For instance, in the liver cells, the process of autophagy was stalled at the step of autophagosome-lysosome fusion. The primary reason behind this failure was found to be the increased level of calcium in the cell due to lipotoxicity. The increased lipids in the cell membrane compromise the action of calcium channels in the membrane, leading to dysregulation in autophagy. This mechanism of autophagic flux inhibition is termed calcium-dependent mechanism of inhibition.

Lipotoxicity and obesity can induce the expression of a special inhibitory protein called Rubicon. This protein functions to inhibit the fusion between autophagosomes and lysosome in a calcium-independent mechanism of autophagic flux inhibition.

The cells of the kidney do not show errors in the step of autophagosome-lysosome fusion under obesity-related stresses. They display another mechanism of inhibition of autophagic flux and display a defect in the lysosomal acidification. The optimum pH of the lysosome is essential for its normal functions and degradative abilities. The increased acidification of lysosomal enzymes can lead to impairment of the cargo degradation process, which is the essence of autophagy. Lipotoxicity can impair the degradative or catabolic abilities of autophagy and thus decrease the autophagic flux in kidney cells.

In pancreatic beta cells, both types of defects in the autophagy processes have been observed under obesity stresses. The failure of autophagosome-lysosome fusion and acidification of lysosomes were both detected after lipotoxic insults. Thus, the autophagy inhibitory mechanisms of lipotoxicity that decrease the autophagic flux vary with tissues and cell types.

Role of Autophagy in Obesity-Related Pathologies

The complex and intricate relationship between the process of autophagy and obesity suggest that autophagy plays a critical role in the regulation of the different pathologies related to obesity. As we know, obesity can have various complications and pathologies which can lead to increased lipid content in cells, accumulation of aggregates of damaged proteins and can cause harm to mitochondrial function. All the pathological effects of autophagy are also a primary substrate of the autophagic process. In this way, autophagy can govern the extent of pathological effects of obesity on the body and can determine the level of complications caused by obesity-related stresses in the body. And the failure or termination of the autophagic process can lead to acceleration in the obesity-associated pathologies in several organs.

Genetic studies have shown that the loss of autophagy genes in liver cells tend to have similar phenotypic effects as observed in obesity-associated non-alcoholic steatohepatitis (NASH). These pathological indications include the formation of protein inclusion bodies, accumulation of fat and liver injury. These findings suggest that obesity and autophagy are strongly interrelated, and that pathologies related to obesity can worsen in cells with defective autophagic machinery. It has been reported that the systemic reduction in the activity of the autophagic process due to the Atg7 gene insufficiency can accelerate the progression of diabetic pathologies in obese individuals. So, the presence of genetic defects in the autophagic system in obese individuals is related to high rates of morbidity and mortality.

However, the over expression of the Atg5 gene, which functions to increase the process of autophagy, has a protective effect on mice against age-associated obesity and insulin resistance. The over expression of Atg7 gene in liver cells showed an improvement in the obesity-associated ER stress. These findings confirm the protective role of autophagy in the body against obesity-related pathologies.

Various therapeutic approaches have been developed to manipulate the process of autophagy to gain benefits for obesity-related pathologies and stresses. For instance, autophagy flux is increased in liver cells by treatment with autophagy-inducing compounds such as carbamazepine and rapamycin. These compounds induce autophagy and help in the catabolic removal of accumulated fats from the liver cells and aid in the healing of injury to the liver. Various calcium blockers are used to restore the autophagic flux in liver cells of obese individuals. These compounds also showed promising results in normalizing the levels of fats and insulin resistance in cases of obesity caused by the consumption of a high-fat diet.

The genetic removal of Rubicon can lead to the restoration of autophagosome-lysosome fusion during obesity-related lipotoxic effects. This restoration of the autophagic process leads to the catabolic removal of accumulated fats from the cell and rids the cell of the toxic effects of obesity. These findings suggest that autophagy provides protection against obesity-related pathologies in liver cells.

However, there are certain studies that suggest the opposite role of autophagy in the determination of obesity-related pathologies in the body. Knockout studies of the Atg7 gene in mice liver and skeletal muscle cells resulted in positive effects on various pathologies related to obesity. These include insulin resistance, adipogenesis, and accumulation of fat. The reason behind these effects upon termination of autophagy is attributed to the synthesis of a special metabolic protein, FGF21, that carries out the metabolism of accumulated lipids in a tissue-specific manner. In similar findings, mice with deletion of the FIP200 gene that is essential for the formation of autophagosomes in the liver cells showed decreased levels of hepatic injury in obese individuals.

These findings suggest a very interesting role of autophagy in the homeostasis of the body and especially in pathologies related to obesity. They show that the process of autophagy plays an important role in controlling the pathological stresses of obesity, but in certain conditions, these stresses overcome the efficiency of autophagy and make it more harmful rather than beneficial for the cell. On the other hand, the complete termination of the autophagic process due to lipotoxic stress can lead to the induction of other compensatory mechanisms that cannot be compromised by the obesity-associated stresses. This process can successfully protect the cells from the complication of obesity and autophagy malfunction. So, in certain cells types, there is a failsafe mechanism that operates in the cell when the process of autophagy has been compromised by the lipotoxic and other stresses induced by obesity.

Autophagy plays an important role in the modification of the pathological outcome of obesity in the macrophages of hepatic stellate cells. The absence of autophagy in these macrophages can lead to an increase in inflammation. Autophagy plays an important role in maintaining the health of the vascular system and inhibition of autophagy due to obesity can lead to a major cardiovascular pathology known as atherosclerosis. Autophagy mediates the process of inflammation in the immune cells and functions to reduce obesity-associated inflammation and other pathologies.

On the other hand, the inhibition of autophagy in hepatic stellate cells leads to a decrease in fibrosis and injury of liver tissue. The inhibition of autophagy in beta cells leads to loss of function and triggers various diabetes-related symptoms, including increased blood sugar level and glucose intolerance, as the cells lose their ability to produce insulin. This condition is worsened in cases of obesity and lipotoxicity as the process of autophagy is hindered and the level of glucose in the blood rises without any check and control. One of the major causes of dysfunction of beta cells and related pathologies is the damage caused by the increased ER stress. In this way, obesity and its related stresses can target and destroy the beta cells of the pancreas and can trigger or aggravate diabetes and other metabolic pathologies.

The ablation of the autophagic process in adipose tissues tends to have beneficial effects against obesity. The process of adipogenesis is dependent on autophagy and the halt in the autophagic process due to obesity also decreases the adipogenic processes. This reduces the potential of an individual to gain a high amount of weight in obesity. So, loss of autophagy in adipose tissues is not so bad for obese individuals and acts as a protective mechanism against gaining extra weight.

Moreover, autophagy carries out the whitening of adipose tissue. The reduction in the number of mitochondria in the adipose tissue leads to the whitening of these tissues and is carried out via autophagic degradation of mitochondria. The decrease of autophagy allows the retention of mitochondria in white adipose tissues those results in an increase in the energy expenditure that consequently leads to the reduction of body weight.

The role of autophagy in each tissue is distinct, and the effect of obesity on the process of autophagy is also different. In some tissues, obesity and related stresses lead to the inactivation of the autophagic process, while in others, obesity leads to the induction of autophagy. The autophagic suppression in skeletal muscle, adipose tissues and liver, can have beneficial effects in obesity and related stresses.

Role of Autophagy in Increasing Lifespan

The presence of biomarkers of aging including increased oxidative stress, damaged mitochondria and other organelles, and loss of membrane fluidity determine the quality of life and longevity. Lifestyle, diet, and exercise can detox our body of aging biomarkers and autophagy is the underlying mechanism of this cellular cleansing.

There are three primary ways to which the cytoprotective effects of autophagy is attributed; these include:

- The buffering of cellular stress according to the availability of nutrients by enhancing the provision of substrates for anabolic reactions and generation of energy to meet the needs of cellular metabolism,

- The removal of abnormal and harmful organelles, including uncoupled mitochondria, therefore removing oxidative stress from the cell, and

- The clearance of aggregates that are potentially toxic proteins.

These cytoprotective effects are regulated and enhanced by various cellular processes and immunogenic responses that help the body improve its functionality and achieve longevity. There are various autophagy-related genes that are related to longevity. The best-characterized pathway is the insulin/insulin-like growth factor 1 (IGF-1) pathway. This pathway includes other vital players of autophagy, including tyrosine kinase receptor, PtdIns 3-kinase and Akt/PKB.

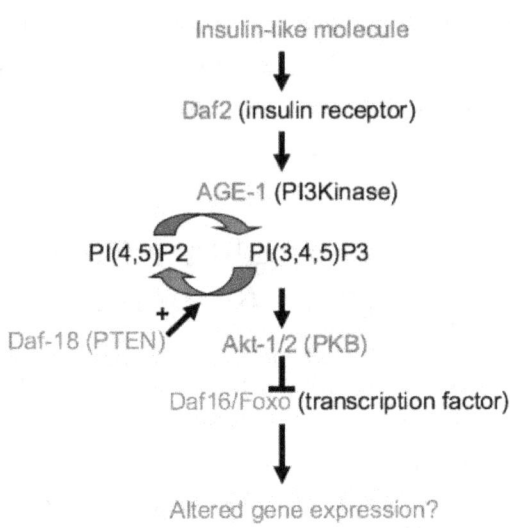

Figure 4. IGF-1 pathway

The longevity studies in nematode, *Caenorhabditis elegans*, suggests that the down-regulation of this cascade has positive effects on the longevity of worms - their lifespan was increased up to three hundred-fold. The inactivation of the IGF-1 pathway induces heat and oxidative stress resistance in these worm, which was found to be the contributing factor in increasing their lifespan. As we already know that Akt/PKB controls the functions of Tor, a suppressor of autophagy, the downregulation of Akt/PKB pathway in this experiment induces autophagy. It can be therefore concluded that autophagy has a significant role in the extension of lifespans.

As we age, there is a subsequent decrease in the process of autophagy which suggests that the two processes are correlated. Primarily, autophagy functions to protect the cell from oxidative damage by removing damaged mitochondria and facilitates other processes like replacement and repair of damaged DNA, lipids, and proteins. All these autophagy-related processes contribute to longevity and life-span expansion.

Mechanisms That Facilitate the Pro-Survival Attribute of Autophagy

Autophagy is a simple process that involves the degradation and removal of unwanted proteins and organelles from the body. The diverse cytoprotective effects of autophagy that lead to an increased life-span and healthy metabolism are attributed to the following processes:

- Proteostasis (Removal of abnormal proteins)
- Programmed cell death (Apoptosis)
- Inflammation
- Metabolism

- Hormesis

Proteostasis

The primary cytoprotective function of autophagy is its ability to remove toxic aggregates of protein that accumulate with aging. Various neurodegenerative disorders that are related to the process of aging, such as Parkinson's diseases and Alzheimer's disease (AD), are found to be caused by the accumulation of defective protein aggregates.

Unlike other processes that function to remove and eliminate defective proteins from the cell, autophagy can degrade large-sized protein aggregates.

Metabolism

Autophagy plays an essential role in various metabolic processes of the body. For instance, autophagy is involved in the lipid homeostasis of the body where it degrades lipid droplets present in cells. This process is known as lipophagy. Autophagy is involved in the process of gluconeogenesis that occurs in the liver where it regulates the level of glucose in the body. It also regulates the process of beta-oxidation of fatty acids and provides an alternative source of energy for the body when carbohydrates and glucose are absent or present in low amounts.

Programmed Cell Death

Activation of autophagy also mediates the process of programmed cell death, or apoptosis. Apoptosis is the regulator of cellular quality, and Beclin-1 mediates crosstalk with apoptotic machinery. This interaction ensures that there is no unnecessary removal of a cell when the damage within the cell can be cleared with autophagy. In this way, damaged mitochondria are removed from the cell, especially those comprising neuronal and muscle tissues, through the process of autophagy with no cellular loss by apoptosis. In this way, autophagy maintains the muscle mass of and neuron number in the body and provides protective effects on the skeletal muscle and nervous system.

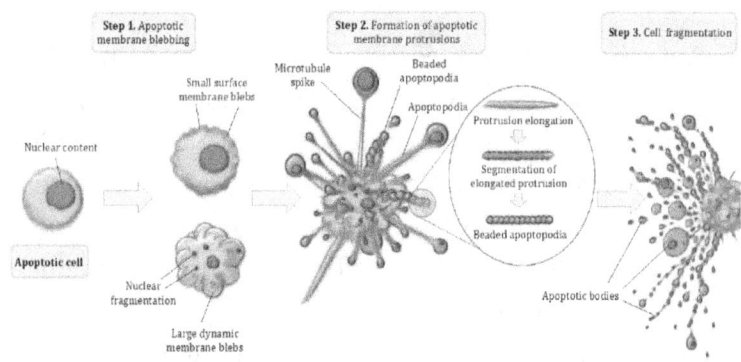

Figure 5. Apoptosis

Hormesis

A widely-studied phenomenon in toxicology is how the presence of a drug or a compound in lesser amounts is more beneficial and less toxic than in high amounts.

Autophagy renders protective effects on the cell by carrying out detoxification and removes reactive oxygen species (ROS) that makes the cell more resistant to stresses that are related to age such as protein aggregates and oxidative damage.

Inflammation

The fact that cells become more inflamed with age has led to the development of a new term known as *inflammaging*. Autophagy plays a vital role in the elimination of inflammation from a cell. The production of pro-inflammatory cytokines in the leukocytes is reduced by the process of autophagy. Autophagy clears the cell from aging markers and ultimately reduces the inflammation from the body.

The Process of Aging and its Link with Autophagy

Aging is one of the strongest natural processes. It is characterized by a progressive decline in the repair and maintenance pathways that are integral to cellular homeostasis. The loss of cellular homeostasis leads to the accumulation of abnormal and dysfunctional organelles and biomolecules. These aberrant cellular components are misfolded, oxidized, aggregated and cross-linked, and have toxic effects on the cell structure and function. These defective molecules can interfere with the cell's functions directly or can compromise the functionality of other molecules and organelles, leading to detrimental effects on the cell. The homeostasis of cellular function is vital for the optimum functions of organs and organ systems. A progressive decrease in the efficacy of cellular homeostasis occurs as we age, leading to various diseases and eventually death.

Over the past century, however, our understanding of the biology of aging has increased. By way of advancements in the field of molecular biology, we have successfully explored the underlying molecular events of the aging process. Interestingly, it has been found that the rate of aging can be controlled by altering certain conserved cellular processes and signaling pathways in various organisms. These findings suggest that the process of aging can be utilized and manipulated as a therapeutic tool to combat various chronic and metabolic age-related disorders.

The processes and cellular pathways that have been found to modulate aging are conserved in various organisms, from yeasts to higher mammals, and have been collectively termed as conserved longevity paradigms. These paradigms will be discussed in the next section.

Conserved Longevity Paradigms in Various Models

Recently, various genes have been identified that control the metabolic functions that influence the aging process in various model organisms. These models include the budding yeast, nematodes, fruit fly, and rodent models. The first studies were carried out in worms and showed that the positive effects of certain mutations in phosphoinositide

3-kinase (PI3K) and insulin/IGF-1–like receptors result in the extension of the organism's lifespan. There are more than 150 *C. elegans* genes that have been found to be involved in increasing their lifespan. And interestingly, most of these genes are part of metabolic signaling and endocrine processes.

The most important and widely studied longevity-associated pathways that primarily control metabolism and nutrient sensing are the insulin/IGF-1 and mTOR signaling cascades. The processes that affect the process of aging include dietary restriction, reproductive system signals and mitochondrial respiration. The list of processes and pathways which modulate aging and their effects on the process of autophagy are given in Table 7.

Table7. List of conserved longevity paradigms in relation with autophagy.

Sr #	Cellular Process	Changes	Effect on Autophagy	Effect on Longevity
1	Insulin/IGF-1 pathway	Decrease in insulin/IGF-1	Increase	Increase
2	mTOR signaling	Decrease in signaling	Increase	Increase

		cascade			
3	Signals from reproductive system	Removal of germline	Increase	Increase
4	Mitochondrial respiration	Reduction in respiration rate	Increase	Increase
5	Dietary Restriction	Applying	Increase	Increase

The signaling cascades and processes that modulate the aging process, directly or indirectly, influence the process of autophagy. The involvement of these processes in regulation of autophagy and longevity make them a desirable candidate for research and provide insight into the complex process of aging. The longevity paradigms that are conserved in all eukaryotic organisms, from yeasts to humans are given below:

- Reduced TOR signaling
- Reduced insulin/IGF-1 signaling
- Germline removal

- Dietary Restriction
- Reduced mitochondrial respiration

Insulin/IGF-1 Signaling

Insulin/IGF-1 signaling is the primary pathway for the regulation of nutritional status in various animals. It plays an important role in the growth of organisms. The hormone insulin (or insulin-like growth factor; IGF-1) interacts with its receptor to activate a cascade of kinases and phosphatases. These include PI3K, and AKT that lead to the inhibition of the transcription factor FOXO. This transcription factor is involved in the stress-coping mechanism of the body and helps the organism to survive under unfavorable conditions.

The downregulation of insulin/IGF-1 in flies, worms, and mice has been found to be linked with an expansion of lifespan. Recent studies have shown that one genetic trait that was found to be common among long-lived humans, ie., centenarians, was the presence of gene mutations in the insulin/IGF-1 pathway. Hence, there exists an interesting relationship between the insulin/IGF-1 pathway and the process of aging – a relationship which is highly conserved.

TOR signaling

The TOR pathway regulates the process of aging. It is the member of the TOR PI3K-related kinase family. TOR is a nutrient-dependent pathway that is activated when a cell has enough nutrients and its metabolism is shifted towards cell division and growth. There are two forms of

TOR complexes, TORC1 and TORC2. These complexes carry out distinct functions in the body by regulating various effector pathways. They mediate nutrient-based and mitogenic signals that carry out proliferation of the cell and determine the cell size. Inhibition of TORC1 has been found to be associated with aging delay. It is activated through the kinase AKT in the presence of amino acids.

The involvement of kinase AKT is a commonality between the insulin/IGF-1 and the TOR pathways. TORC1 leads to the activation of multiple anabolic processes. These include biogenesis of ribosome, initiation of translation, transport of nutrients, and inhibition of autophagy.

TOR signaling regulates the process of aging in many organisms. A reduction in the TOR activity can prolong the lifespan in yeast, flies, worms, and mice. There are two main processes that are influenced by TOR that effect longevity which are:

- Ribosomal protein S6 kinase (S6K) acts as a downstream target of TOR. The inhibition of S6K leads to the reduction of protein synthesis that leads to expansion of lifespan in worms, yeast, flies, and mice.

- TOR regulates the cellular recycling process of autophagy which mediates longevity.

Dietary restriction

Dietary restriction involves cutting down on nutrients while avoiding being malnourished. This approach is considered as the most robust methods that are currently being used to delay aging. This method has shown promising results in extending the lifespan of mice, hamsters, fish, yeast, invertebrates and apes. Advances in molecular biology have led to the findings that highlight the role of nutrient pathways, TOR signaling and insulin/IGF-1 in contributing to the longevity effects of dietary restriction.

Signals From the Reproductive System

Interestingly, there exists an inverse relationship exist between fertility and lifespan. Research shows that certain signals from the reproductive system have a positive effect on lifespan. By removing germ cells or germ line precursor cells from worms and flies, the lifespan of flies and worms were extended. However, the removal of the complete reproductive system or sterility did not have an effect of longevity which suggests that lifespan extension is not related to sterility but rather, the absence of signals which promote aging from germ line cells.

Reduced Mitochondrial Respiration

One of the most widely studied hallmarks of aging is the free-radical theory. The fact that the level of free radicals in the body is increased as we age can be one of the most obvious reasons for the cellular and organ dysfunction that is related to aging. Reactive oxygen species (ROS) can cause molecular damage to cells and cell components and can have deleterious effects on the body. One of the most important organelle of the cell, the mitochondria, plays an important role in the determination of ROS levels in the cell. ROS is produced during mitochondrial respiration and the reduction of mitochondrial respiration and reduced electron transport chain function can decrease the levels of ROS and increase lifespans in worms, yeast, flies, and mice. Studies in worms show that an increase in longevity is mediated by an upregulation of the mitochondrial unfolded protein response (UPR).

Aging is controlled in a highly conserved manner by various signaling pathways and processes. The primary objective in aging research is to find out whether these signaling pathways and processes that control lifespan have a common downstream mechanism. Current evidence suggests that autophagy, which is the cellular recycling process, is one of such mechanisms. Autophagy maintains cellular homeostasis and plays an important role in cleansing the cell from signs of aging and disease. In doing so, it helps in increasing the organism's lifespan.

ROLE OF AUTOPHAGY IN THE BODY

The process of autophagy occurs in a systematic manner in the body with varying rates in different parts and tissues of the body. As each organ of the body has different metabolic needs, the rate of autophagy also varies in each organ. The organs where the most efficient and elaborate system of autophagy occurs are the brain, liver, and muscles. Autophagy plays a different role in each of these organs and ensures the functioning, survival, and development of the cells of these tissues. The role of autophagy in these organs is distinct and will be discussed in the next section.

Autophagy and the Brain

As we know, autophagy is the primary housekeeping process of the cell. It can remove and recycle aged proteins, protein aggregates, and entire organelles. The most widely studied role of autophagy is in the brain cells where it provides remarkable neuroprotective effects.

Protein aggregates or inclusion bodies are common hallmarks of age-related neurodegenerative disorders. There is increasing evidence that these aggregates have toxic effects on the brain cells and interfere with neuronal function. These aggregates affect the hampering of axonal transport, integration of synapsis, regulation of transcription in neuronal cells, and mitochondrial function in the neurons, which lead to dysregulation of neuronal activity.

Neuroscientists have been focusing their research to find an effective treatment for neurodegenerative diseases to slow the age-related neural loss down and find way ways to clear the protein aggregates from neurons. Various studies imply that loss of autophagy increases the formation of inclusion body and triggers a neurodegenerative cascade. These findings highlight the role of autophagy as a built-in defense mechanism to cleanse the brain and nerve cells from inclusion bodies. It is becoming increasingly important to develop a better understanding of autophagy to better control the factors that influence healthy aging and neurodegeneration as well as to facilitate the development of new drugs and treatments.

Role of Autophagy in the Neurons

Various studies suggest that autophagy plays an important role in preventing the accumulation of inclusion bodies in the brain cells and renders a neuroprotective effect. The relationship between neuronal pathology and autophagy has been established by studying the effects of knockout mutations of the Atg5 and Atg7 genes in neuronal cells in mice. These genes are vital for the formation of autophagosomes and are therefore critical for the autophagic process. Deletion of these genes leads to increased cell death, progressive deficits in motor activity, and increases the formation of inclusion bodies. This shows that the loss of autophagy is enough to trigger a neurodegenerative cascade that compromises brain functions.

Mice with brain-specific Atg7 knock-out mutations showed an increased mortality rate, reduction in body size, loss of movement coordination and tremors, which are an indication of neurological faults. Lack of autophagy leads to neuronal loss; the most damaging type of neuronal loss is known as gliosis. Gliosis is characterized by the loss of pyramidal neurons, which is a diagnostic marker of neurodegenerative events.

The increase in age of Atg7- and Atg5-deficient mice led to an increase in ubiquitin-containing inclusion bodies in their neurons. The lack of autophagy was likely the reason for the formation and accumulation of inclusion bodies as normal autophagy functions to remove protein aggregates from the cell.

Neurodegenerative pathogenesis of brain-specific Atg5-deficient mice has been studied. These mice suffered from severe motor deficits, loss of Purkinje cells that regulate coordination and movement and accumulation of inclusion bodies. All these findings show that autophagy has a crucial role in the homeostasis and functioning of neurons. The optimal functioning of the autophagic system ensures the brain health, improves cognition, delay age-related memory loss and protects the brain from neurodegenerative diseases.

Autophagy and Successful Brain Aging

Thus far, we have established the importance of autophagy in preserving the health of the brain and nervous system. But there is also a definitive role of diet and calorie restriction in the protection of brain functions which can be attributed to the neuronal autophagic flux. Evidence from around 70 years of research on the link between calorie-restriction and autophagy provides fascinating insights on the role of CR-induced neuronal autophagy that protects the brain and increases the lifespan of humans. Therefore, following a low-calorie diet either by intermittent fasting or a fat-rich diet in combination with autophagy-inducing dietary supplements can significantly contributes to successful and healthy brain aging.

Autophagy and Liver

The self-eating process of autophagy plays an important role in the normal functioning of the liver. This catabolic pathway contributes to maintaining the homeostasis of the liver by regulating the energy needs of the cell as well as facilitating the removal of damaged organelles, misfolded proteins and droplets of lipids. In this way, autophagy has a major impact on hepatocytes. Other cells of the liver where autophagy plays an essential role include the hepatic stellate cells, endothelial cells and macrophages. Autophagy is a vital process for the health and proper functioning of the liver and any kind of error or abnormality in this process can lead to liver damage and dysfunction, which can also cause various diseases.

The most common type of liver diseases that occur due to the faulty autophagic system includes various storage diseases. As the liver is the metabolic hub of the body, it acts as a reservoir for different kind of metabolites. The inability to degrade and remove these metabolites from the liver cells due to malfunctioning of autophagy can cause the over-accumulation of these compounds in the cells of the liver and trigger various storage diseases. The most common types of liver diseases include Wilson's disease and alpha-1 antitrypsin deficiency. Several other kinds of liver disorders many also arise due to defects in autophagy; these include non-alcoholic steatohepatitis, hepatic carcinoma, chronic alcohol-related liver disease and acute injury of the liver tissues. The detrimental effects of autophagic errors make the process of autophagy a potential therapeutic strategy as by manipulating the process of autophagy and modulating its beneficial effects on the cell, we may be able to treat various liver diseases.

As discussed earlier, the liver is the primary metabolic and detoxifying organ in the body. As autophagy plays a significant role in the cleansing and cleaning process of cells, it ought to have a significant role in the liver. Apart from removing aggregates of abnormal proteins and damaged mitochondria, autophagy is also involved in the removal of swelling in hepatocytes.

A major inducer of liver autophagy is starvation. The major physiological functions of autophagy in the liver include β-oxidation of fatty acids, regulation of metabolic pathways such as gluconeogenesis and the formation of ketone bodies. Gluconeogenesis requires amino acids that are provided by degradation of proteins through the process of autophagy. The production of fatty acids is carried out mainly through the autophagic degradation of triglycerides that are stored in the form of lipid droplets. Autophagy regulates the level of very low-density lipoprotein (VLDL) particles in the serum through the process of lipophagy. This results in the release of fatty acids into the blood. Additionally, the autophagy process also plays an essential role in the maintenance of plasma glucose levels in neonates during starvation and fasting. Autophagy in the hepatocytes also provides protection against accumulation of fat in the liver.

Hepatoprotective Properties of Autophagy

Autophagy in the liver cells imparts an overall protective effect by providing protection against various kinds of stresses and diseases. Studies involving mice models with defective autophagy pathways are more vulnerable to liver injury from different toxic agents including alcohol, ischemia-reperfusion, and high levels of toxic free fatty acids. Macroautophagy protects against the death of liver cells by eliminating misfolded proteins, oxidized lipids, damaged mitochondria, and oxidative stress. It can provide the cells with the necessary nutrients to maintain cellular energy needs under conditions of injury and stress.

Autophagy and Hepatic Stellate Cells;

Jekyll or Hyde for the Liver?

Hepatic stellate cells (HSC) are a type of mesenchymal cells that are present in the liver. They are located between the hepatocytes and blood vessels. HSCs are characterized by the presence of droplets of lipids and thin protrusions that extend around the blood vessels in the liver. HSCs play important roles in the physiology and fibrogenesis of the liver. Fibrogenesis of the liver is a cellular response to chronic liver injury. This can result from various metabolic disorders, alcohol consumption, or presence of chronic viral infections. Unlike the positive effects of autophagy on other liver cells, HSCs are prone to certain harmful effects of autophagy which can lead to liver damage and fibrosis. Autophagy is considered as a deleterious pathway in these fibrogenic cells.

It has been identified as the key player in the phenotypic switch of hepatic stellate cells from normal to fibrogenic phenotype as it causes a progressive loss of lipid droplets that contain retinoid. Catabolic action of autophagy degrades the lipids droplets via lipophagy. An increase in the catabolism of retinyl esters by autophagy leads to the generation of free fatty acids. These free fatty acids lead to the increased production of ATP, which acts as a trigger for the HSCs to acquire the fibrogenic profile. An increase in autophagic flux and the number of autophagic vacuoles in liver cells have been associated with an increase in LC3-II in human HSCs, proving the role of autophagy in inducing the fibrogenic activity of HSCs. Fibrosis of the liver tissue leads to chronic liver damage and loss of liver functions. It has been found that the primary triggers for the upregulation of autophagy in HSCs are ER and oxidative stress.

Various clinical interventions involving the inhibition of autophagy have resulted in the reduction of fibrogenic effects of HSCs. Inhibition of autophagy downregulates the fibrogenic properties of HSCs, which includes a reduction in cell proliferation rates and a reduced expression of fibrogenic genes. By using therapeutic measures, such as downregulation of the Atg5 or Atg7 genes, or by reducing oxidative stress, we can minimize the risks of liver fibrosis by the action of hepatic stellate cells. In this way, autophagy acts as a two-way sword for the liver cells, and it becomes a tricky question of whether it is the Jekyll or Hyde for the hepatocytes. Regardless, the importance of autophagy for the normal functioning and homeostasis of the liver is unquestionable.

Autophagy in the liver is an interesting process as apart from HSCs, it has positive effects on other types of liver cells including hepatocytes and macrophages. In fact, renders a hepatoprotective effect. While the death of a hepatocyte triggers the fibrogenic profile of HSCs, the process of autophagy prevents this trigger and protects the cell from fibrosis. Interestingly, in cases of α-1 antitrypsin deficiency, the induction of autophagy provides protection against hepatocyte death and fibrosis of the liver tissue. In epithelial cells, the process of autophagy proves to be a protective pathway against damage and fibrosis in various organs, including liver and kidneys. Thus, we can conclude that autophagy acts as a friend for macrophages and hepatocytes.

Autophagy and Liver Regeneration

The liver is a special organ as it can regenerate itself and heal. Autophagy plays an important role in liver regeneration. It carries out the elimination of damaged proteins from the liver and maintains cellular energy needs; both these processes are crucial for tissue regeneration. The role of autophagy in elimination of damaged proteins and maintenance of intracellular energy highlights its importance in the process of liver regeneration.

Only a few studies have analyzed the role of autophagy in the regenerative process. It has been found that the removal of a small part of the liver led to an induction of autophagy in the early stages of the regeneration process.

Knockout mice with a specific deletion in the Atg5 or Atg7 genes in liver cells suffered from the accumulation of abnormal mitochondria and an impaired ability of liver regeneration when exposed to liver tissue removal. Hepatocytes with an abnormal autophagic system are unable to maintain the energy level that is required for cellular physiology and become aged. Macroautophagy provides protection against various defects in the regeneration process that may occur due to chronic liver injury.

Autophagy and Muscles

The skeletal muscles and neuronal tissues are the main sites of autophagy as the muscle cells contain the highest number of mitochondria and require an efficient system of organelle turnover. However, increased autophagy in muscle cells also makes them more prone to damage if any kind of abnormality arises in the process of autophagy.

Various muscular disorders have been linked with the abnormal accumulation of autophagic vacuoles. This group of muscular dysfunction is termed as autophagic vascular myopathies (AVMs). Two of the main disorders that affect humans due to errors in the autophagy system are Pompe disease and Danon disease. They are discussed below.

Danon Disease and Pompe Disease

The autophagic pathway plays a very important role in the homeostasis of the skeletal muscles. It provides a cellular quality-check system that ensures the degradation of proteins and removal of old organelles. The autophagosomes function to engulf damaged organelles, cytoplasm and protein aggregates. This autophagosome then attaches to lysosomes for the degradation of its cargo. Lysosomes are an important part of the autophagic process and any kind of dysfunction in the lysosomal role in autophagy can have serious health effects. The importance of lysosomes in the muscle is highlighted by the important role it plays in a group of muscular diseases. These disorders are caused by the accumulation of autophagic vacuoles in the cell due to impaired lysosomal function.

The accumulation of autophagosomes proves to be toxic to the cell and hinders the normal cell physiology and function. This group of disorders is referred to as autophagic vacuolar myopathies (AVMs). These include Danon disease (DD), Pompe/glycogen storage disease type II (GSDII) and X-linked myopathy with excessive autophagy (XMEA).

Danon disease is an X-linked dominant disease. It is characterized by an anomaly of lysosome-associated membrane protein 2 (LAMP2). Patients with DD suffer from cardiomyopathy, weakness of muscles and mental retardation. LAMP2 carries out the maturation of autophagosomes and aids in the process of endosomal fusion. A lack of this gene causes failure of autophagosomal fusion to the lysosome, which results in accumulation of these autophagic vesicles in the muscle cells. This leads to muscular weakness and deterioration of mental health.

Pompe disease is characterized by deficiency of lysosomal enzyme known as acid alpha-glucosidase. The deficiency of this enzyme causes abnormality in the degradation and removal of glycogen. The accumulation of glycogen occurs in various tissues, however, the most harmful effects have been observed in the skeletal and cardiac muscles.

Autophagy and the Vascular System

Like in other cells and tissues, autophagy plays a protective role in vascular endothelial cells that are prevalent in our veins and arteries. In the vascular endothelial cells, autophagy carries out a crucial role by providing protection against various pathophysiological stimuli. These include exposure to reactive oxygen species, hypoxia, end products of glycation, oxidized low-density lipoprotein, and lipopolysaccharides. Various natural compounds that have antioxidant and anti-inflammatory activity, such as vitamin D, curcumin, and resveratrol, can promote autophagy in ECs. The use of these compounds helps to protect against oxidative stress and endothelial inflammation and injury.

Autophagy in Atherosclerosis

Atherosclerosis is a chronic disease of the arteries. It is characterized by inflammation of the arterial wall and has high mortality rates all over the world, and especially in developing countries. Atherosclerosis occurs due to the production and accumulation of lipid-containing plaques in the vessel wall. It is one of the most prevalent age-related diseases. Other risk factors that lead to an increased risk of developing atherosclerosis include hypertension, smoking, obesity, diabetes and hypercholesterolemia.

Recent evidence suggests that the presence of a dysfunctional autophagic system is the primary cause of atherosclerosis. The vascular cells fail to trigger autophagy when they are exposed to oxidative stress, cytokines and oxidized lipids that are present in plaque. This tends to have a damaging effect on vascular health as the presence of plaque leads to hardening of arteries and a loss of elasticity. As autophagy is a catabolic process, the formation of atherosclerotic plaque should be solved by this process. However, defects in autophagy lead to the failure of removal of plaques from the arteries and it has therefore been postulated that autophagy plays a main role in modulation of atherogenesis and in the stability of atherosclerotic plaque. It has been found that defective autophagy promotes the process of cell death and apoptosis in macrophages. It promotes premature senescence in vascular smooth muscle cells (VSMCs) and both apoptosis and senescence in epithelial cells. By developing a better understating of the defects of the autophagic process in these three types of cells, we can model the autophagic process for therapeutic purposes and find new autophagy-based cures for vascular diseases.

Methods to Monitor Autophagy

Several methods have been developed to monitor and measure the rate and flux of autophagy in cells. These methods have become widely used and have gained great importance owing to the significance of autophagy in the field of research and therapeutic sciences. Recent advancements in microscopic and molecular biology have led to the development of various methods that have high accuracy. Some of the widely used methods for the measurement and monitoring of autophagy are discussed below:

1) Staining Methods and Microscopy

- Monod-ansylcadaverine (MDC)
- LysoTracker
- Acridine orange

2) Screening of autophagic markers and immunohistochemistry

- LC3

3) Autophagic flux

- Sequestration assay
- Use of radio labeled assay
- Ape1 (aminopeptidase 1) maturation assay

1). Staining Methods and Microscopy

The acidotropic stains, including MDC (Monodansylcadaverine), LysoTracker and acridine orangeare commonly used for the labeling of acidic compartments in cells. These include autolysosomes, endosomes, and lysosomes. An increase in these organelles can be easily monitored by using these stains and subsequent visualization through electron microscopy. As membranes are easily stained by these acidotropic stains, the double-membrane of autophagosomes are proven to be the most prominent structures for monitoring the rate and level of autophagy in any cell.

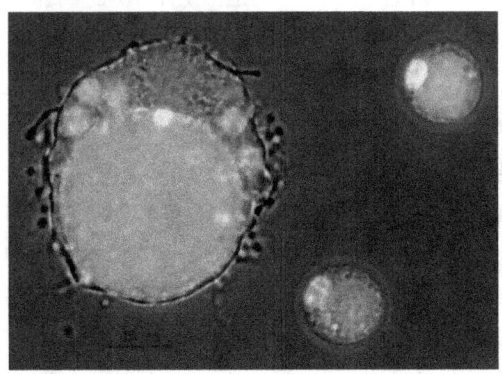

Figure 6. Lysotracker stain

2) Screening of Autophagic Markers and Immunohistochemistry

Another method for the detection of the level of autophagy in a cell includes screening for the presence of certain autophagy-related proteins or autophagic markers. One of the most widely used proteins is a homolog of Atg8 in yeast, termed as LC3. LC3 is a microtubule-associated protein and is one of the most efficient autophagy markers. The level of LC3 in a cell is equivalent to its level of autophagic processes. There are two predominant forms of LC3 protein in the cell, LC3-II and LC3-I. The level of LC3-I is typically high in normal cells, while LC3-II levels are only increased in a cell during autophagy. The relative changes of LC3-II and I provide a clear indication of the autophagy levels in a cell.

There are two ways through which the level of LC3-I and LC3-II levels and their interchangeability is analyzed to monitor the level of autophagy. These include western blotting and immunofluorescence or immunohistochemistry. During western blotting, the level of LC3-II in the cell can be visualized on a gel using cell extracts and a suitable marker for the protein. For immunological analysis, antibodies against LC3-II can be used for detecting the level of autophagy marker in a cell. Another method is the fluorescence methods, where fusion of a fluorescent marker to the N-terminus of LC3 can be used to monitor the sub-cellular localization of this protein and thereby, the induction of autophagy in a cell.

These methods are used to determine the steady-state measurements of autophagy in the cell. To determine the efficiency of the autophagy process in certain cells and at specific conditions, it is necessary to use other methods which can measure the autophagic flux. Autophagic flux is determined by analyzing the rate of lysosomal delivery of the cargo and its degradation in the lysosome. This is a vital feature of the autophagy process and its analysis aids us in determining the factors which affect the process of autophagy.

3) Autophagic flux

There are different methods that can be used to monitor autophagic flux. Sequestration assay is one of the most widely used methods for this purpose. In this method, an artificial cargo, [3H]-raffinose, is injected into the cytoplasm of the cell. This cargo is sequestered and transferred into an insoluble fraction through the formation of autophagosome. The rate at which [3H]-raffinose is transferred to autophagic vesicles and removed from the cytoplasm is monitored and autophagic flux is determined.

Another method to monitor the autophagic flux is by analyzing the rate of protein degradation. This method involves the use of radiolabeled proteins. The degradation of proteins into amino acids will result in the release of radioactive amino acids into the cytoplasm. The level of radioactivity will be proportional to the rate of protein degradation by autophagy.

The Ape1 (aminopeptidase 1) maturation assay is also used to determine the autophagic flux in the yeast cell. It involves the autophagic conversion of Ape1 into its mature form in the autophagic vacuoles that are equivalent to the lysosome in mammalian cells.

Other strategies to measure autophagic flux include the monitoring of turnover of LC3-II, or the removal of autophagic substrates from the cell.

WHEN DO THE RESULTS OF AUTOPHAGY START TO SHOW?

Autophagy is a highly regulated and complex process. To get the full benefits of this process, it is important that we adopt a certain routine and then follow it strictly. By following a strict autophagic routine, one can start seeing the results of autophagy in around two weeks.

In one study, based on finding the positive effects of autophagy, they determined the level of health biomarkers, such as skin complexion, body/mass index (BMI) etc., in the body. It was found that by eating certain autophagy inducing foods and following an exercise routine for eight weeks, the individuals felt more active, energetic and healthy.

As autophagy is induced in response to stressful conditions, one must trick his body into believing there is stress. The study used the following key autophagy-activators that function perfectly to induce stress in the body:

- Low-carb and high-fat diet
- Excluding proteins completely from the diet

- Fasting for two days a week or trying other types of intermittent fasting
- Doing high-intensity interval training exercises

Autophagy—The Best Body Detox Regimen

If you need a detox, you don't always have to go with liquid kale and other stuff that doesn't taste good. Autophagy is a natural way through which our body cleanses itself. It helps in maintaining the quality of cells and its organelles, reduces inflammation, and keeps your body running in tip-top shape. Autophagy is essentially a fine-tuning mechanism or the housekeeping staff of our body.

Autophagy and intermittent fasting together provide the perfect detox regimen. They help to clear our body of harmful toxins, burn extra weight, and renew our body right at the molecular level. The detoxification effects of autophagy and intermittent fasting are amazing. Together they promote the anti-aging process and lead to longevity.

PRECAUTIONS RELATED TO AUTOPHGY

Autophagy is an amazing process that has many beneficial effects on the body. However, to enjoy the benefits of autophagy to the fullest, it is necessary to follow the authentic and safe methods of inducing autophagy.

While practicing fasting to induce autophagy, it is advisable to fast with good and healthy intervals, rather than long-term fasting.

If you are suffering from certain health problems and are using medications for it, it is advisable to consult with a doctor before adopting any autophagy-related routine, such as fasting, high-intensity exercising or dietary restrictions. People suffering from hypoglycemia, hypertension or diabetes, or those with a family history of these diseases, must take precautions before going for autophagy inducing routines. Women who are pregnant or are breastfeeding infants must not try intermittent fasting. If you are a beginner to fasting, it is advisable to start with a relatively easy approach called crescendo fasting which involves a 12-hour fast routine.

Autophagy

If you are opting for calorie restriction as an inducer of autophagy, then it is advisable that you keep a complete check on your diet and make sure all the essential macro and micronutrients are included in the diet. This will ensure a balanced diet and will protect you from malnutrition.

While doing high intensity exercises, we should take care and listen to our body. One should not push himself beyond his limits and should allow his muscles and body to heal and repair before exercising again. It is also advisable to follow recommendations from a professional trainer.

So, the takeaway message is that it is necessary to stay safe while aiming to achieve certain goals with autophagy. Autophagy has a lot to offer for the betterment and well being of our health, but there are certain notions and protocols that we should follow to avoid any kind of undesired outcomes.

Melany Flores

Future Perspectives Regarding Autophagy and Its Therapeutic Role

The Unanswered Questions

The relationship between food and autophagy has increased the importance of nutrition and dietary choices. Furthermore, the role of dietary modifications in disease prevention has become increasingly important. Various health-promoting dietary components and their mechanism of action on the physiology of the body have been identified and their effects on autophagy have been widely studied. Autophagy is upregulated by consuming certain foods and has been used as a key therapeutic tool for the treatment of neurodegenerative diseases and cancer. However, the exact role of dietary components in the regulation of autophagy and autophagic flux and the diverse effects of autophagy in the body needs to be further investigated. Moreover, the exact role of autophagy in cancer needs more extensive research as multiple studies suggest that under certain circumstances, autophagy acts as a suppressor of tumorous cells, while in others it aggravates the tumor. It is necessary to determine when autophagy is beneficial and when it is non-beneficial, so that we can effectively manipulate the autophagic process and develop autophagy-inducing drugs for improving human health. There are some unanswered questions regarding the autophagic process in relation to dietary components that may govern its effectiveness in therapeutic field. For instance:

1. Where, when and how are the autophagy-inducing food components metabolized in the cell?

2. Will the nutrients survive in the human body in an active form for long enough to affect the autophagic process?

3. Will the metabolites of these nutrients also be biologically active or have the potential to influence autophagy?

4. What should be the effective and safe concentration of these nutrients that one needs to consume to trigger autophagy?

5. Will the effect of these food components be systematic or targeted? Will the nutrients only interact and affect the cells of the gastrointestinal tract, or will they be able to enter the blood and reach other parts of the body?

6. Is it necessary to prepare, store, and consume the food in a specific manner to obtain their autophagic benefits?

7. What kind of interactions will these compounds have with pharmaceutical drugs?

It is important to identify every compound that is present in the foods we eat and understand their effects on the body. It is also important to understand how all the components present in our diet could affect autophagy and other cellular processes. If we use dietary components and food supplements that induce autophagy for therapeutic purposes, it is necessary that we understand the interaction of food components with each other as well as their overall effects on the body. For example, if we use the autophagy-inducing diet for treating breast cancer, we should be able to make a solid hypothesis about the effects of such a diet on the hormone levels in the body. Such diverse implications of diet, governed by physiology as well as genetics, makes autophagy-induced therapy a tricky matter. We should utilize methods such as personalized-therapy and nutritional-healing so that we can get the most out of the autophagic process for therapeutic purposes.

CONCLUSION AND FINAL THOUGHTS

Autophagy was initially identified as a responder of cellular stress, but with increasing research and studies it has been established that it is a much more complex and beneficial process of the mammalian physiology. Autophagy plays an important role in the maintenance of normal physiological roles and contributes to regulating the development, growth, and aging of mammals. It is the natural cleansing process of the cell and rids the body of signs of aging and disease.

Autophagy plays a significant role in a variety of disorders and diseases. It is a complex process, and its exact role in various diseases remains controversial. As we age, the process of autophagy gradually diminishes, which is manifested by a decrease in the formation of autophagosomes or the inappropriate fusion of these vacuoles with the lysosomes. In the case of neurodegenerative disorders, the accumulation of certain proteins is attributed to the failure in the autophagic elimination of these toxic proteins. Various lysosomal disorders are attributed to the dysfunction of the autophagic process that leads to the accumulation of lipid droplets in the lysosomes. Autophagy plays a very confusing role in cancer, where it acts as tumor suppressor in the initial stages but as a tumor promoter by protecting the cancer cells from the immune system. Moreover, autophagy positively and negatively regulates various kinds of muscular and heart disorders respectively. On the other hand, the induction of the autophagic pathway plays an important role in fighting and removing foreign pathogens. It is a vital part of innate immunity. The effect of downregulation of autophagy in obesity and related stresses varies and is highly tissue-dependent.

Autophagy operates locally and systematically in various tissues of the body. It is involved in the development and growth of tissues in different ways. When autophagy is impaired, the differentiating tissues undergo deleterious effects and the whole physiology of the body is disturbed. Autophagic errors lead to various metabolic and chronic disorders as well as cancers, which can be life-threatening.

Various regimens have been adopted to artificially induce autophagy in the body. These approaches help in the upregulation of autophagy to gain benefits like anti-aging, detox, weight loss, and longevity. It also provides protection against neurodegenerative diseases, chronic illnesses, diabetes, hypertension and cardiovascular diseases.

Further research is required to understand the systemic role of autophagy in the mammalian life cycle. This will provide us with a better understanding of developmental biology in relation to the process of autophagy, which will aid us in finding new targets for the treatment of complex and chronic diseases. We need to utilize the basic scientific knowledge that we have about autophagy for therapeutic purposes. Because of the extremely diverse role of autophagy in biochemical and signaling pathways, its importance is greatly increased from a clinical perspective. The role of autophagy in the manifestation of metabolic disorders, neurodegenerative diseases, aging, inflammatory diseases and cancer have made it an ideal candidate to be explored for its therapeutic and diagnostic implications in managing various diseases.

I hope this book provided you with all the useful information that you wanted to have. Don't forget to write a short review of the book on Amazon if you liked it!

***

www.ingramcontent.com/pod-product-compliance
Lightning Source LLC
Chambersburg PA
CBHW060846220526
45466CB00003B/1256